'What happens when the consulting room meets the courtroom and both face the street? Rakesh Shukla brings half a century of democratic politics, forty-five years in the Indian legal profession and a lifetime's engagement with psychoanalysis to bear on the urgent questions of our times. Moving between tribal district magistrates' courts and the Supreme Court of India, between the clinic and the protest site, this stunning book asks what Freud's boldest ambitions so long buried under professional respectability might still offer a society riven by communal violence, caste oppression, gender crime and the creeping advance of authoritarian nationalism.

Drawing on Klein and Bion, on Reich and Marcuse, on Sanskrit love poetry and Hindi cinema, on the myths of Ravana and the trauma of Partition, Shukla illuminates the unconscious forces at work in courtroom judgments, in intimate violence, in the manufactured hatred of designated "enemy" communities and in the psychic roots of fascism. He brings a psychoanalytic lens to honour killings and public lynching, to the biases of judges trained to believe themselves impartial, to the devastating mismatch between trauma's effects on memory and the law's demand for coherent narrative.

This book is a tour de force about the cost of keeping psychoanalysis insular and the extraordinary possibilities that open up when it is not. Bravo!'

- **David Morgan**, Chair of Political Mind, Training Analyst and Supervisor, British Psychoanalytic Association, Fellow of the British Psychoanalytic Society, Editor of *The Unconscious in Social and Political Life*

'Rakesh Shukla is a lawyer and a psychoanalyst of rare distinction, with professional experience in courts in several cities in India, which includes long-time discussions with judges and studies of potential influences of human unconscious in the usual practice of law.

With his solid contributions as a consultant to the International Psychoanalytical Association (IPA) Committee of Psychoanalysis and Law of the International Psychoanalytical Association, Mr. Shukla also carries this question to a global stage, enriching it with his vast professional experience.

Out of decades of practice across multiple instances of the Indian judiciary, and his intimacy with the courtrooms, corridors, chambers where law lives, his work with judges, besides his psychoanalytical understanding of the human mind, he invites us in this book on a groundbreaking journey across the multiple intersections between law and the unconscious, between objectivity and the subjective bias that can inhabit law around the world, particularly, of course, in India

Courageous as well as sensible, this is a book for our times, exploring forces that pulse beneath the surface of human beings, also delving into the inner world of judges and confronting authoritarianism and the very foundations of democracy.

It is a seminal work. A necessary voice. It is a must-read for professionals and lay people who want a closer understanding of the relation between law, the human soul and society.'

- **Plinio Montagna**, Author, Professor, Psychiatrist and Psychoanalyst, Former President, Brazilian Psychoanalytic Society of São Paulo, Former President, Psychodrama Society of São Paulo, Former Editor, *Brazilian Journal of Psychoanalysis*, Professor, Euro-Latin America Psychosomatics School, Professor, Psychoanalytic Psychosomatics Group of Moscow, Russia, Former Chair and Present Consultant International Psychoanalytical Committee on Psychoanalysis and Law

'In *Psychology, Law and Society in India: The Unconscious Republic*, Rakesh Shukla offers a penetrating exploration of the hidden psychological forces that shape Indian society, its laws, and its institutions. Moving from intimate relationships to communal conflict, from the courtroom to the inner world of judges, this book reveals how love, rage, trauma, prejudice, masculinity, and authority continue to influence public life in ways often unrecognized.

Bringing psychoanalysis into conversation with law, politics, and everyday experience, Shukla asks difficult but urgent questions: What drives ordinary people toward violence? How do memory and trauma enter legal testimony? Why do societies create divisions between "us" and "them"? And what unconscious impulses lie behind the making and interpretation of law?

Provocative, interdisciplinary, and deeply relevant to contemporary India, this book invites readers to confront the unseen republic within.'

- **Dr Ronald Doctor**, Training Analyst and Fellow of the British Psychoanalytic Society, Fellow of the Royal College of Psychiatrists, Chair of the IPA Psychoanalysis and Law Committee and Hon. Lecturer, University College London

Psychology, Law and Society in India

Psychology, Law and Society in India: The Unconscious Republic uses psychoanalysis to look below the surface of the apparently rational legal system, consider the subterranean factors at play and devise interventions to bring law closer to justice.

With specific reference to India, Rakesh Shukla takes a look at the relationship between love and rage in intimate relationships, the impact of the father-son dynamic in politics and inter-community relations. Shukla considers the dynamics behind parental love and 'honor killings', Hindu sexuality and fanaticism, and how the 'other' comes to be viewed as 'evil'.

Grounded in law, clinical practice and interventions in judicial training, this book will be of interest to anyone wishing to learn more about the interface of society, the psyche and law.

Rakesh Shukla engages with the complex interface of law, society and psychology, conducts workshops with judges on minimizing impact of biases, prejudices and stereotypes on the judicial decision-making process. Rakesh has designed and taught courses on law and psychology.

Titles in this series

Violence or Dialogue? Psychoanalytic Insights on Terror and Terrorism
Sverre Varvin

Pluralism and Unity? Methods of Research in Psychoanalysis
Jorge Canestri

Truth, Reality and the Psychoanalyst: Latin American Contributions to Psychoanalysis
Silvia Flechner

The Geography of Meanings: Psychoanalytic Perspectives on Place, Space, Land, and Dislocation
Salman Akhtar

Linking, Alliances, and Shared Space: Groups and the Psychoanalyst
Rene Kaes

Children in Genocide: Extreme Traumatization and Affect Regulation
Suzanne Kaplan

Resonance of Suffering: Countertransference in Non-Neurotic Structures
Andre Green

The First Dictionary of Psychoanalysis: A Gift for Sigmund Freud's 80th Birthday
Richard Sterba

The Letters of Sigmund Freud to Jeanne Lampl-de Groot, 1921-1939: Psychoanalysis and Politics in the Interwar Years
Edited by Gertie Bögels

Winnicott's Letter to Bion: Playing, Dreaming, and Beyond
Edited by Steven H. Cooper and Christopher G. Lovett

Psychology, Law and Society in India

The Unconscious Republic

Rakesh Shukla

Routledge
Taylor & Francis Group
LONDON AND NEW YORK

Designed cover image: Getty Images

First published 2027
by Routledge
4 Park Square, Milton Park, Abingdon, Oxon OX14 4RN

and by Routledge
605 Third Avenue, New York, NY 10158

Routledge is an imprint of the Taylor & Francis Group, an informa business

British Library Cataloguing-in-Publication Data
A catalogue record for this book is available from the British Library

ISBN: 9781041040941 (hbk)
ISBN: 9781041040927 (pbk)
ISBN: 9781003626794 (ebk)

DOI: 10.4324/9781003626794

Typeset in Palatino
by KnowledgeWorks Global Ltd.

To our indomitable strivings for an equal, just and harmonious society

Contents

Foreword

With stunning modesty Mr. Rakesh Shukla, a lawyer and a psychoanalyst, offers what he calls a 'minor contribution' to a psychoanalysis of law and national life events. This modesty, like law itself, thus revels in what has been termed 'narcissism of small differences'. But as you read this magnificent narrative, you will realize that law and psychoanalysis is an important genre and sphere inaugurated here. Mr. Shukla commands an advantageous position being a legal practitioner and a minuscule band of therapists.

As Salam, A., Shanker, A., & Verma, M. (2022) say: 'while psychoanalysis 'has been around in India for over a century now, beginning with the works of G.S. Bose in 1910s… the popularity, acceptability and accessibility of Psychoanalytic Psychotherapy has had a fluctuating course in the mental health arena of the country. The initial enthusiasm seems to have been circumscribed within the academic community and appears to have taken objections with its 'foreign origin and roots'. This approach to psychotherapy was seen as 'alien to the Indian culture and was not welcome warmly as a treatment strategy'.[1]

One welcomes, however, especially in times of global turbulence, this slender but extremely significant work – a guide to sanity (which must be described as abnormal normality). The very title of this book – the 'Unconscious Republic' – speaks volumes, especially at the time of celebration of the 75th anniversary of the Constitution of India. It brings to us live what Fredrick Jamieson termed 'political unconscious'[2] where he explicated the political dimension of creative works' – a text is a 'socially symbolic act' where the "political unconscious functions as a destabilizing force revealing the disjunction between a text's explicit meaning and the 'buried reality' of class struggle."

The learned author recalls the trauma of the Partition, and in this he places himself second only to the illustrious author of ancestral treatise on constitution law by Shri H.M. Seervai.[3] But Mr. Shukla goes further in recalling the relationship between trauma and monuments. Shukla's wry lament about the great Taj Mahal is worth noting: 'The Taj Mahal in Agra is one of the Seven Wonders of the World, built in the memory of the Queen Mumtaz Mahal by Emperor Shah Jahan. Lurking behind the beauty of the monument of love is the stark reality that Mumtaz Mahal died of postpartum haemorrhage while giving birth to their fourteenth child'. One wishes he explores, more fully in future, the relation between beauty, justice and pain, which Sigmund Freud broadly articulated is a relation between the drives of Eros and Thanatos (life and death instincts), respectively, though a recent essay suggests a non-dualistic approach.[4]

Turning from monuments to official courtroom linguistic flourishes, his experiential and comparative observation is striking: 'the whimsical nature of the human psyche is nevertheless on full display....[in] the individual adorning the bench going off in irrelevant, tangential directions'. Lawyers have little option but to follow the whimsies of the judge with quaint phrases like 'I bow to what has fallen from your Lordship's lips'. 'In India the English of the England of the 19th and early 20th Century still enjoys currency', even when in 'the home country of the language the United Kingdom there have been commissions to simplify legal language'. Indeed, a 'large amount of mental space, time and energy of an advocate is spent in figuring out the psychology of the judge to put the submissions in the most appealing way'. In part, Shukla says, this 'led me to psychoanalysis– rather than figuring out the mindset of judges, time and effort channelized to ordinary individuals and therapy seemed more meaningful'.

He notes that the 'impact of the ubiquitous caste system with its rigid stratification of superiority and purity by birth, with the lowest rung considered as "untouchables," on the 'working of laws' is immense and 'Judges trying cases under anti-discriminatory laws bring to bear all their rationality and logic, yet we see the unconscious biases reflected in the judgments', especially concerning the 'gender crimes like rape and sati'. In saying this, Shukla reinforces the great Dr. Ambedkar on the systemic discrimination against India's *atisudras* (the social and economic Dalit have-nots) and holds a warring mirror to civil society and the State in India.

The learned author reminds us that 'the formula of picking up a historical trauma acting as if it happened yesterday and conflating the perpetrators at the time with the present targeted community ... reflects a phenomenon that has played out in other parts of the world as well'. He especially mentions the bombing of Hiroshima and Nagasaki that was 'preceded by the depiction during World War II of the "enemy" Japanese as sub-human, barbaric, blood thirsty vermin' and the ways in which Slobodan Milosevic 'picked up the defeat of Serbia in 1389 and conflated the present-day Bosnian Muslims with Ottoman Turks who were victorious in the Battle of Kosovo, whipping up fury that led to ethnic cleansing in 1995'.

Here we enter, what Jaques Derrida called the 'a founding act of violence that is neither legal nor illegal but establishes the very system of legality'. The law's authority stems from 'mystical' foundational act, somehow self-justifying itself, without any legal 'precedent' to justify it pre-exists! Thus, the authority of law is not rational but relies on this foundational violence to maintain itself.[5]

Such cruel human, and human rights, violations occur all too frequently and value of linking law, whether national or international, to the theory and practice of psychoanalyses is immense. Mr. Shukla traces how Indian constitutional development has been haunted by this originary trauma in all its practices of governance, development, rights and justice.

It has been said (by Georges Gurvitch, one of the forerunners of the European sociology of law) that a 'little law takes us away from sociology but too much of it leads us back to it'. By 'little law', he signified law merely as an apparatus of the technicalities of law but 'more law' represents social, economic and ideological contexts, even pre-contexts, in which it comes into operation. And what Gurvtich thus said about the law is also true of psychoanalysis and law as well. The learned author rightly says: 'in making meaning of these subterranean feelings, emotions and perspectives that underlie broader social and political happenings' psychoanalysis provides 'a unique lens, with deep focus as well as a panorama view…'.

Some readers may feel provoked by what gets said in the book, but its main purpose is not any foolish/unstudied partisan political outburst of sentiment. Rather, the learned author prompts further a constitutional quest for a more equitable world, free from prejudices and illusions, and always geared to the freedom, justice, equality and fellow feeling implicit, and at times explicit, in a democratic, republican and socialist constitution.

Verily, to this end, psychoanalysis provides a new commonsense to constitutionalism in India. Mr. Shukla reminds us that in India, the independence 'movement led by the Congress Party was centred on issues of land reform and striving for a more egalitarian society'. Paradoxically, this political passion for social change 'rather than battling social oppressions in the outer world' led to "adjusting" the inner world of the individual to accept the myriad injustices of the world we inhabit. I think that the description of 'political passion for change' sums the overall aspiration and endeavour of this work.

Upendra Baxi
Emeritus Professor of Law
University of Warwick and Delhi

Notes

1 See, their 'Psychoanalysis in India: A Story of Ascent, Decline and Revival'. *Psychoanalytic Psychotherapy*, 36(4), 300–311.
2 Fredrick Jamieson, *The Political Unconscious: Narrative as a Socially Symbolic Act* (London, Routledge, 1981).
3 H.M. Seervai, Constitutional *Law of India* (In three Volumes (4th Edition. Lucknow, Eastern Book Co, 4th edition, 2023).
4 Maria Kli, 'Eros and Thanatos: A Nondualist Interpretation: The Dynamic of Drives in Personal and Civilizational Development from Freud to Marcuse', *The Psychoanalytic Review*, 105:1:67–89 (2018). She engages the 'unfolding of the dynamic of drives within the individual's psychic development and the civilization process'.
5 Peter Fitzpatrick develops this there brilliantly in his *The Mythology of Modern Law* (London, Routledge (1992).

Series Editor's Foreword

The International Psychoanalytic Association Publications Committee is honoured to present a new book from the *International Psychoanalysis Library series*. The focus of the Library is on today's scientific developments throughout the IPA, with an emphasis within the discipline on clinical, technical and theoretical advances, as well as on empirical, conceptual and historical research projects. The Publications Committee of the International Psychoanalytical Association is pleased to present the new book, *Psychology, Law and Society in India: The Unconscious Republic,* authored by Rakesh Shukla.

The book is grounded in the perspective that psychoanalysis can offer insights as we grapple with socio-political issues of our times. The author reflects that psychoanalysis offers valuable insights into contemporary issues in India, particularly regarding individual and collective violence such as hate crimes, lynching, communal violence, honour killings and domestic abuse.

The author shares some remarkable information about the Indian Psychoanalytical Society, which was established in 1924, with its headquarters in Kolkata – the epicentre of social movements for egalitarian change in India – and had little to do with the social concerns of the times. From his point of view, psychoanalysis stayed in its isolated esoteric corner and made the process of training to be an analyst extremely cumbersome and inaccessible. Following independence from British rule, India moved towards a more egalitarian society in which socialism and communism became mainstream ideologies, in contrast to post-WWII (World War II) America. Psychoanalysis in India has not addressed caste, class or gender inequalities, and exploring this gap is beyond the scope of this book. The use of the criminal justice system to crush democratic, peaceful movements demanding legal rights was incontrovertible. The author also states that many legal systems mistakenly believe judges are immune to community bias and always deliver impartial justice. Unconscious partisanship influenced his interest in law and psychoanalysis.

The first chapter, "Of Gods and Demons: The Murderous Impulses of the Ordinary," examines humanity's desire for clear-cut notions of good and evil, acknowledging that reality is far more complex. It discusses how both notorious villains and everyday individuals can blur the line between hero and villain, and explores what fuels such extremes in human beings.

The second chapter, titled Love and Rage in Intimate Relations: Sorties in Narcissism and Projection, examines how oral traditions, media and popular culture shape our ideas of love and affect our behaviour through a psychoanalytic perspective, helping us understand their influence on the human mind.

The third chapter is titled "Law and Psychoanalysis: The Logical meets the Irrational". In contrast to the logical and the rational, the human psyche is like a seething cauldron of fears and anxieties, insecurities and prejudices, as well as raging contradictory emotions like love and hate, empathy and cruelty. The chapter also explores how extralegal factors, such as judges' intuitions, often regarded as indicators of truth, may actually reflect biases and prejudices in the courtroom.

The fourth chapter is titled "Trauma and Testimony: Memory, Psyche and the Demands of Law", examines how trauma is often misunderstood by judges and highlights the limitations of laws designed for individual crimes when applied to collective offenses like public lynching or targeted killings. It discusses how collective trauma can cause inconsistent testimonies, leading to witnesses being deemed unreliable or even convicted of perjury. The trauma of the legal process on the victim-survivor is explored with special emphasis on crimes against children.

The fifth chapter is titled "Inner World of Judges: Psychoanalytical Explorations" provides an account of the framework of the interventions, using a methodology that gives primacy to 'affect' and 'free association' in the training sessions.

The penultimate chapter is titled ""Us" and "Them": The Psychology of Inter-Community Relations," attempts to look beneath the surface at the intra- and inter-psychic processes at play in the raging tensions and conflicts among various communities in India. It examines the application of the formula for picking up a historical trauma, acting as if it happened yesterday, and conflating the perpetrators at the time with the present targeted community.

The final chapter examines how male sexuality intersects with fascist ideologies in India, particularly the push for uniformity under "One Nation, One Language, One Leader, One Food, One Religion." Drawing on Reich's theory that sexual repression fosters obedience to authority, the chapter outlines cultural values like celibacy and myths about sacrificing virility, exploring their role in making individuals susceptible to reactionary ideologies. It also considers how reverence for the Mother-Goddess and related anxieties contribute to demonizing certain communities and analyses the projection of shameful feelings onto others, fueling fears of violation by "enemy" groups. The chapter suggests that collective acknowledgement of these projected emotions could help counteract such processes.

The book also addresses ancient and contemporary cultural challenges in India, offering an opportunity to delve into psychoanalytic engagement with law, historical trauma, and intra- and inter-psychic trauma. This new book is a resource for psychoanalysts, historians and philosophers to understand, from a new perspective, some of India's conflicting issues.

Silvia Flechner
Series Editor
Chair, IPA Publications Committee

Preface

In *Psychology, Law and Society in India: The Unconscious Republic*, Rakesh Shukla brings together half a century of engagement with democratic left politics and more than four decades of legal practice to craft an unusually intimate and analytically powerful meditation on how law actually operates in a deeply unequal society. Moving from small magistrates' courts in tribal-dominated districts to the highest court of the land, Shukla traces how caste, class, gender and communal biases seep into the everyday functioning of the criminal justice system, despite its formal commitment to the "Rule of Law" rather than the "Rule of Men."

At the heart of the book is a simple yet far-reaching proposition: psychoanalysis, long confined to the individual clinic and to elite metropolitan circles, should be reclaimed as a critical tool for understanding the socio-political crises of our time. Shukla argues that in India, psychoanalysis largely "stayed in its isolated esoteric corner," structurally unreachable to the poor and disconnected from struggles against caste, class and gender oppression, though social movements and the freedom struggle ignited expectations of egalitarian transformation.

Against this backdrop, *The Unconscious Republic* holds that psychoanalytic thinking can illuminate some of the most troubling phenomena of contemporary India: public lynchings, "honour" killings, communal violence, domestic violence and the daily humiliation set in caste hierarchies. The opening chapters explore what Shukla calls brutal "*impulses of the ordinary,*" laying spectacular outbreaks of violence within a wider projection, splitting and disavowal through which communities offload their shame, rage and aggression onto constructed "others."

One of the book's most distinctive contributions is in its sustained attempt to read legal institutions psychoanalytically. In a series of vivid courtroom vignettes and careful readings of doctrine, Shukla shows how judges' "gut feelings," anxieties about national disintegration, and unconscious identifications with a threatened "motherland" shape the adjudication of sedition, anti-terror, morality and narcotics laws, often to the detriment of presumptions of innocence and civil liberties. A striking early episode describes a Supreme Court judge trembling with barely contained fury in a wildlife conservation case, as arguments about roads, detonators and "left-wing extremism" tap into fantasies of being beheaded by mobs and swallowed by anarchy – fears that are nowhere acknowledged in the written judgment, yet palpably structure the hearing.

From here, the book develops a rich inquiry into the "inner world of judges," interrogating the legal fiction that appointment to the bench somehow washes away the prejudices, stereotypes and social locations that all of us "imbibe in an osmosis-like process." Shukla draws on his experience of conducting affect-focused workshops with members of the higher judiciary, where free association and the exploration of "us" and "them" narratives help surface unconscious caste and class assumptions. These chapters challenge readers to reconsider cherished ideals of neutrality and objectivity, without lapsing into cynicism about the possibility of justice.

The later sections widen the lens to examine the psychology of inter-community relations and the rise of authoritarian, majoritarian politics. In a compelling psychoanalytic reading of Indian fascism, Shukla explores how myths of sons surrendering virility to fathers, the valorization of celibacy and the deification of the Mother Goddess interact with anxieties about emasculation and pollution. These cultural configurations, he suggests, predispose segments of the male psyche to seek refuge in ideologies promising One Nation, One Language, One Leader and a purified community cleansed of "rapacious" enemy males.

In one of the book's most unsettling and illuminating passages, Shukla juxtaposes the destruction of the Somnath temple in 1025, the demolition of the Babri Masjid, the genocidal campaigns in Bosnia and the depiction of the Japanese during the Second World War to show how political weaponization of historical sufferings occurs dissolving medieval invaders into present-day minorities to approve contemporary violence. The book here draws on global histories of genocide, racism and xenophobia to demonstrate that the Indian "unconscious republic" is part of a wider, disturbing pattern.

Yet, this is not a counsel of despair. Throughout, Shukla is attentive to the constructive potential of psychoanalytic work when it moves beyond the consulting room. He points towards collective processes through which communities might "take back" disowned feelings of dirt, lust and aggression, rather than endlessly projecting them onto demonized others; he sketches how trauma testimony, especially of survivors of sexual and caste-based violence, could be received by courts in ways that recognize complex post-traumatic responses rather than punishing them.

Psychology, Law and Society in India: The Unconscious Republic will speak to lawyers, judges, psychoanalysts, social scientists and activists who sense that something vital is missing from purely doctrinal or purely sociological accounts of law's violence and law's promise. Drawing on Freud and Kakar as much as on constitutional jurisprudence, human rights reports and case law, Shukla offers a rare, genre-defying work that is at once memoir, theoretical reflection and a call to reimagine how societies might confront their own unconscious.

Rejecting both technocratic complacency and apocalyptic resignation, this book offers a lucid and unsettling account of how the hidden life of the psyche shapes law, politics and everyday cruelty in modern India—and how, in carefully listening to that hidden life, one might yet glimpse the possibility of a more equitable world.

Justice S. Ravindra Bhat (Retired), Supreme Court of India
Chairperson, National Task Force on Student Mental Health and Suicide Prevention in Higher Educational Institutions
Chair Professor M.K. Nambiar Centre for SAARC
Comparative Law Centre, NALSAR Hyderabad

Acknowledgements

I would like to acknowledge Deen Dayal for his consistent friendship over the decades. A number of ideas in the book surfaced in an incipient form over innumerable walks during our college days. Conversations with close friends Jogin, Laxmi, Shifa, Dilip, Kishwar, Arunesh, Sumita, Shamim, Anurag, Jyotika, Ayesha and numerous others helped evolve concepts that have found words in this book. Involvement with democratic movements for change and interaction with comrades in labour, Adivasi, civil rights and feminist movements enabled me to keep my feet firmly on the ground while working in small ways to build a better world.

I am grateful to friends and colleagues in the legal community, Murali and Ravi, who in their subsequent avatars as Justices S. Muralidhar and S. Ravindra Bhat fully endorsed the idea of psychological intervention in judicial training. I am indebted to Prof. Ved Kumari who took on board the importance of psychoanalytical intervention in judicial training and as Chair of the Delhi Judicial Academy facilitated my conducting training programmes. I am grateful to Prof. Sri Krishna Deva Rao, a pioneer in legal education, who readily agreed to introduce a Seminar/Clinical course on the Psychology and Law at the National Law University Odisha.

I owe a special thanks to Mallika, my Training Analyst, and my music teacher, the dhrupad singer Nirmalya De, for my developing the ability to accept the tedious and persevere in creative undertakings. I think with pleasure of the late Stuart Twemlow, founding co-editor of the International Journal of Applied Psychoanalytic Studies (IJAPS) and Douglas Kirsner, Professor, Deakin University. The friendship started on their visit to India and continued over the years and their appreciation and recognition of my writings has meant much to me. I would like to acknowledge and thank Nadia Ramzy, founding co-editor of IJAPS, for her consistent appreciation of my writings. I wish to specially acknowledge writer-psychoanalyst the late Sudhir Kakar who opened up the area of the impact of popular culture on the psyche and was consistently supportive of my forays into taking the psychoanalytic frame into diverse areas.

I would like to thank Joseph for help in conceptualizing the book for publishing. I am grateful to Susannah and Eleanor for the seamless coordination and guidance in the process of bringing the book to publication. I thank Uday for his tech help. In addition to the constant sharing and evolving of ideas, I am deeply grateful to Laxmi for the transformation of messy convolutions into readability.

I would like to acknowledge and thank my daughters Rakhee and Priya whose support contributed to an ecosystem conducive to writing. Last, but not least, I would like to acknowledge the role of and thank the poet and writer, Raksha, my mother.

Consent for publication: Written consent was obtained for the material used from the cases of two clients in this publication.

Introduction

Social movements for egalitarian change and the justice delivery legal system might seem worlds apart from contemporary psychoanalysis. But from where I stand, they are closely intertwined. I come from half-a-century of involvement with democratic left politics and about 45 years in the legal profession, having practiced in courts in different parts of the country, from lower courts in tribal dominated districts to the highest court of the land in India's capital.

An autobiographical piece, "Of the Bar, the Bench, the Couch, the Flag and Anxious 'Love',"[1] attempts to draw together the varied elements of my winding journey, traversing courts, clinics, protest sites and inter-personal relationships. The present book is an attempt to fill in the skin and bones, the blood and gore, the anxieties and fears, the troubles and tribulations, the joys and doubts, the certainties and uncertainties of human existence that I have encountered. I am often greeted with puzzled astonishment in my new *Avatar* as a psychoanalyst.

Perhaps, the astonishment speaks of the sanitization of psychoanalysis, a somewhat blinkered containment of Freud to the clinic, inured from the audacious leaps of "The Future of an Illusion" and "Civilization and its discontents." Russel (1983) speaking of the invisibilizing of the vibrant political life and spirit of the second-generation psychoanalysts led by Fenichel, observes "The psychoanalytical profession, however, abandoned Freud's bold theorizing and questioning. Against Freud's profound hopes, psychoanalysis became insular, medical and clinical.... Freud wrote simply and elegantly for a wide cultural audience. ... In a technical and medical prose, contemporary analysts complacently write for one another" (p. xi).

In the context of my retaining a lively curiosity and critical questioning engagement with the world, perhaps, partly, due to lesser feelings of shame about the sexual and not looking upon it as Breuer (1893–1895) observes "something dirtying and besmirching" (p. 219). Freud (1915) makes a case for not excessively suppressing wishful impulses and notes, "It happens to be precisely the components of the *sexual* drive that are specially marked by a capacity for this kind of sublimation, for exchanging their sexual aim for another one which is comparatively remote and socially valuable" (p. 51). Tagirov (2017)

DOI: 10.4324/9781003626794-1

observes "Another theoretician of the repressive hypothesis, G. Marcuse, who understands eros, like late Freud, in an extremely broad sense – as a desire for pleasure, which is not limited only to genital pleasure and even to bodily pleasures at all, but includes, for example, the pleasure of free labour (here the Marxist roots of the theory of Marcuse are obvious), writes about the specific castration to which an individual in a repressive civilization is exposed. Unlike practices of the castration of eunuchs, for example, where the reproductive function is primarily cut off, the suppressed individual is deprived of all eroticism that does not meet the principle of reproduction of the genus." Reich (1942) links suppression of sexuality to repression in the psyche making the individual more susceptible to authoritarian ideologies.[2]

The criticality of engagement, perhaps, meshed in with the incipient beginnings of ambivalences and questioning the neat demarcation of "Heroes" and "Villains"; "God" and "Satan"; "Love" and "Hate" and being drawn to seeking the "hidden from the manifest." The unconscious imbibing from the innumerable myths of deceitful gods and honest demons accompanied by the frisson of exhilaration at the fervour and pomp of Hindu festivals.

In North India, as children, we looked forward with great enthusiasm to the Hindu festival of *Dushera*. The making of an effigy of the ten-headed demon *Ravana* on a bamboo frame stuffed with firecrackers, old newspapers and other inflammables to be slayed by *Rama* was the build up to the grand finale of the enactment of the legend of the epic Ramayana. Paradoxically, *Ravana*, the demon in the legend, is supposed to be a repository of great knowledge of the sacred ancient texts like the *Vedas* and *Shastras*, and a devotee of the god Shiva. Usually, cities and towns in North India have a centralized ground referred to as *Ramlila Maidan* where a grand giant effigy of a ten-headed *Ravana* is erected. In parallel to the grand central celebration, in local neighbourhoods children go house to house asking for donations to build small effigies of *Ravana* in little humble celebrations and there is a live intertwining of the festival with the world of a child. An arrow from *Rama* ignites the flammable configuration accompanied by much cheering at the destruction of the demon.

The meta reading of the child-like imagination of an external ten-headed monster is the vanquishing of the inner demons of *Kama* – Lust, *Krodha* – Anger, *Lobha* – greed, *Mada* – pride, *Maatsyasya* – Envy, *Moha* – Delusion, *Agyan* – Ignorance, *Ahamkara* – grandiose I-self, *Svartha* – Selfishness and *Asakti* – attachment. This seamlessly flows like a confluence of rivers into two stanza couplets of Saint-poets like Kabir and Rahim, which are a part of childhood often have a surface literal meaning and meta deeper truths. Kabir's couplet is illustrative:

> *"Jin dhuna, tin payian ghere pani paith;*
> *main budhi budan dari, rahi kinare baith"*

(trans. 'One who searches and dives into deep waters gets it; I was scared of drowning stayed on the shore")

A literal reading is that the one who dives deep into the water gets the pearl, not the one who sits scared on the shore. This is to be followed by an engagement with the deeper meaning of the couplet with the pearl not to be taken as a precious gem but as a symbolic representation of yearnings as per our inclinations. In a similar vein, stories, folklore, poetry on the anguish of separated lovers but alluding to deeper meanings under the surface.

It is in making meaning of these subterranean feelings, emotions and perspectives that underlie broader social and political happenings that psychoanalysis provides a unique lens, with deep focus as well as a panorama view, so to speak.

The book stems from the perspective that psychoanalysis can offer insights while grappling with socio-political issues of our times. Freud (1921) also engaged with group psychology, but psychoanalysis took a turn to almost exclusive individual therapy in the clinic. Freud (1918) writes "On the other hand, it is possible to foresee that at some time or the other the conscience of society will awake and remind it that the poor man should have as much right to assistance for his mind as he now has to the help offered by life-saving surgery; and that the neuroses threaten public health no less than tuberculosis, and can be left as little as the latter to the impotent care of the individual care of the community" (p. 160).

The Indian Psychoanalytical Society which was established in 1924 with its headquarters in Kolkata - the epicenter of social movements for egalitarian change in India - had little to do with social concerns of the times. In a sense, psychoanalysis stayed in its isolated esoteric corner and made the process of training to be an analyst extremely cumbersome and inaccessible. The Society celebrated a hundred years of existence and has a mere 50 psychoanalysts on its rolls.

In parallel developments, psychoanalysis in the United States seems to have suffered a similar narrowing and constricting fate. Glover (2023) in his Presidential Address, American Psychoanalytic Association, New York, February 3, 2023, titled 'Psychoanalysis—More than a Profession', observes, "The professionalization of psychoanalysis also fostered exclusion, hierarchy, and an orthodoxy that resisted change and led to stagnation and decline. As the profession matured, this self-imposed closure and isolation deprived us of the contributions of outsiders and cross-pollination with other disciplines" (p. 112).

The fleeing of Freud and other psychoanalysts from rising Nazism to Europe and the prevalent McCarthyism in the United States with the concomitant paranoia about "Satanic Communism" seems to have played a role in moving away from a more group- or people-oriented psychoanalysis to a confinement of the profession to the clinic in the West. Glover (2023) observes, "The rise of Nazism led to the mass migration of continental European analysts. They hid their socialist inclinations as they began new lives in countries, such as the United States, where anticommunist sentiment was strong……. Despite its humanitarian ethos and libratory potential, psychoanalysis has mirrored societal inequities." Jacoby (1983) writing of the left oriented émigré psychoanalysts like Fenichel, Edith Jacobson and Annie Reich who had to flee fascism writes, "Initially they buried, adjourned or abandoned a political psychoanalysis in the name of personal survival" (p. 7).

In the context of the lack of appeal of psychoanalysis for individuals striving for a more equitable world, Shukla (2016) observes, "It was the passion for social change and the slotting of psychoanalysis as primarily serving to maintain the status quo. Rather than battling social oppressions in the outer world, 'adjusting' the inner world of the individual to accept the myriad injustices of the world we inhabit." In India, the independence movement led by the Congress Party was centred on issues of land reform and striving for a more egalitarian society. Unlike the post Second World War atmosphere in United States, the prevailing atmosphere with the dawn of independence from British colonial rule was a shift towards a more equal society in India and socialism and communism were accepted and legitimate ideologies. An in-depth analysis of the non-engagement of psychoanalysis in India with the caste, class and gender inequalities in society, despite liberty and freedom in the air, is outside the scope of the present enterprise and requires in-depth research and study. However, this disconnect forms the backdrop of the current book.

The words of Glover (2023), "Psychoanalysis, like liberalism, espouses racial equality but has been content to benefit from its privileged status," may perhaps be a pointer in understanding the total disconnect of psychoanalysis from democratic movements for social change in India. In a similar vein, the words of Jacoby written in the context of psychoanalysis in America seem to ring true in India "Then psychoanalysis seemed very much in tune with the conservative and conformist times. It had become a respectable medical activity with prosperous practitioners and prosperous clients" (p. 6). It is nobody's case that the poor do not have mental health issues; the fee structure of psychoanalysts has made it outside the reach of the vast majority of people in India.

The fulcrum of the book is the belief that psychoanalysis can contribute constructively to the issues of the present times in India. The chapters attempt to bring to bear a psychoanalytical lens to individual as well as collective violence – love and hate crimes, public lynching, communal violence, "honour" killings and domestic violence. My innings in law begin from a small Magistrate's court in a Balod, a town in then Madhya Pradesh, presently the tribal majority state of Chhattisgarh carved out of the larger central province. I was working with an organization of contract workers in iron ore mines and marginal farmers and my work entailed dealing with the criminal cases instituted against workers demanding their rights.

The use of the criminal justice movement to crush democratic peaceful movements demanding legal rights was incontrovertible. The turning of a civil industrial dispute into a 'law and order' problem and the partisan use of the police in favour of the industrialist-owners was in full display. The use of force by the police, baton charges and at times firings as well as arrests in trumped up criminal cases was the order of the day. The exposure to the class bias of the legal system began with a bang so to say. The perils of practicing law in a highly polarized atmosphere of workers' struggles also were brought home.[3] Anyone stepping into a courtroom can observe caste, class, gender and religious biases playing out in the entire legal process. The erroneous assumption that individuals appointed as judges magically become free of the biases and prejudices of their community and administer impartial justice seems to run through all legal systems. By and large, the partisan attitudes at play were unconscious and in a sense drove me to engagement with law and psychoanalysis. The writings are part of a striving for a more equitable society, including a fair and just legal system.

The first chapter, "Gods and Demons: The Murderous Impulses of the Ordinary," explores the human yearning for the simple binaries of "Good" and "Evil" and "God" and "Satan." However, the realities are more complex. The human facets of the "most murderous of villains" and violent-aggressive aspects of ordinary mortals, perhaps blur the neat division into hero and villain. From the doctors who, despite the Hippocratic Oath to do no harm, actively collaborated in horrific experiments on inmates of concentration camps while being caring family men in the evenings, to the next-door-neighbour with a regular middle-class job who beats a maid to death all bear examination and constitute the subject matter of the chapter. What drives human emotion in its extremes?

The quicksilver transformation of love to rage erupting into violence against the "loved" one takes us to the next chapter. The scrutiny of the influences that shape our notions of love ranging from oral traditions to movies and songs and their playing out in the arena of life through a psychoanalytic lens offers some understanding of the impact of popular culture on the human psyche.

My clinical practice over the years has witnessed a considerable amount of time and effort spent in the trials and tribulations of love. As a client evocatively put it in Hindi, "Sir, *main pyar ki gathri khol rahan hun*" ('trans. Sir, I am opening the bundle of love') when nudged by the therapist to "unpack love." Kakar (1989) in the context of the presence of women disillusioned after marriage in therapy clinics notes, "Generally fated for disappointment, the fantasy of constituting a 'couple', not in opposition to the rest of the extended family, but within this wider network, is a dominant theme running through women's lives, actual and fictional." (p. 22). The Taj Mahal in Agra is one of the Seven Wonders of the World, built in the memory of the Queen Mumtaz Mahal by Emperor Shah Jahan.

Lurking behind the beauty of the monument of love is the stark reality that Mumtaz Mahal died of postpartum haemorrhage while giving birth to their 14th child.

The second chapter – "Love and Rage in Intimate Relations: Sorties in Narcissism and Projection" – engages with the influences that shape our notions of love, expectations from lovers and the interplay of reality versus constructed objects of desire. African-American feminist writer bell hooks (1984) makes a case for paying "attention to systems of domination and the inter-relatedness of sex, race, and class oppression" (p. 31) and argues that the "belief that women can achieve equality with men of their class without challenging and changing the cultural basis of group oppression" (p. 20) is fallacious. As hooks (2000) pithily puts it, "There can be no love without justice." It explores to what extent the qualities we perceived in the person we "fall" in love with were present or were a product of our rose-tinted glasses. Freud (1921) notes, "It is even obvious, in many forms of love choice, that the object serves as a substitute for some unattained ego ideal of our own. We love it on account of the perfections which we have striven to reach for our own ego, and which we should now like to procure in this roundabout way as a means of satisfying our narcissism" (p. 104).

The chapter takes a look at tales from ancient Sanskrit texts from 12th to 13th Century, Adventures of Amir Hamza with oral traditions from 7th Century, early written versions in 11th–12th Century and an illustrated 1,400-page version commissioned by Mughal Emperor Akbar in the 16th Century. The continuity of the ancient tales to books with tales of perfidy sold on the pavements of streets in India is testimony to the universality of the theme of love and longing. We make connections with some of the myths of doomed love prevalent across cultures from the colds of Siberia, the Mediterranean Greece to the hot desserts of Arabia and India. The chapter then moves on to legends of love at first sight and tortured star-crossed lovers, driven by anguish and despair popular in India. It traces the influence of Hindi cinema and songs from the 1950s to the present in shaping notions of love, of women, of consent, of wooing, of gender stereotypes impacting intimate heterosexual relationships in India today.

The next section with three chapters engages with the interface of law and psychology.

As we step into the temple of justice set up to administer the "Rule of Law" and not the "Rule of Men," the whimsical nature of the human psyche is nevertheless on full display. We may find the individual adorning the bench going off in irrelevant, tangential directions. Lawyers have little option but to follow the whimsies of the judge with quaint phrases like "I bow to what has fallen from your Lordship's lips." In the home country of the language, the United Kingdom, there have been commissions to simplify legal language, but in India, the English of the England of the 19th and early 20th Century still enjoys currency. A large amount of mental space, time and energy of an advocate is spent in figuring out the psychology of the judge in order to put the submissions in the most appealing way. In part, this led me to psychoanalysis – rather than figuring out the mindset of judges, time and effort channelized to ordinary individuals and therapy seemed more meaningful.

The chapter "Law and Psychoanalysis: The Logical Meets the Irrational" examines the role of the invisible extra-legal factors at play in the court room like the "gut feelings" of the judge popularly trusted in society as being truth indicators, but may be little more than biases and prejudices at play. It tries to illustrate the role of phantasies of protecting the "mother" and "motherland" combined with anxieties about the breaking up of the territory of India, thereby adversely impacting sound legal principles like "presumption of innocence" and the "burden of proof on the prosecution" in cases as well as when adjudicating the constitutionality of sedition and anti-terror laws. Next, we examine the impact of notions of vice and morality of the individual judge in particular cases as well as in cases challenging the constitutionality of the laws in areas like sex work and narcotic and psychotropic drugs on the anvil of unreasonable encroachment of fundamental rights. The framing and the working of laws tackling social malaises like dowry and pre-natal sex determination and sex selective abortion are analysed. The impact of the ubiquitous caste system with its rigid stratification of superiority and purity by birth, with the lowest rung considered as "untouchables," on the working of laws forms a separate section. Judges trying cases under anti-discriminatory laws bring to bear all their rationality and logic, yet we see the unconscious biases reflected in the judgments. The working of the law in gender crimes like rape and sati are scrutinized. The stresses and strains of overworked judges are taken on board and we explore possible avenues to move forward.

Unfortunately, the requirements of law like clear time lines as to events, precision of corroborative detail, logical consistency, and confident answers to questions put in cross-examination, are all at odds with the impact of trauma on the psyche of the survivor. Trauma may evoke a very high degree of anxieties and fears as to the well-being and existence of the survivor leading to panic attacks with somatic symptoms like breathing distress and suffocation, at times leading to a freezing or shutdown. A blurring and fragmentation of memories and sudden flashbacks may take place. The conscious "verbally accessible memory" of trauma is distinguished from the non-conscious impact, which cannot be accessed at will in the context of coherent narratives of events and the answering of questions put by courts and in cross-examination in an adversarial system.

The trauma of the legal process on the victim-survivor is explored with special emphasis on crimes against children. The chapter titled "Trauma and Testimony: Memory, the Psyche and the Demands of Law" focuses on the systemic flaw of the impact of trauma being little understood by judges trained in the rigours of the law and evidentiary requirements. The inadequacy of laws framed for individual crimes in dealing with collective crimes like public lynching and targeted killings based on religion, caste or ethnicity is scrutinized. The dynamics of collective trauma may play out in a blurring and conflation of stories, which comes out as being inconsistent in the repeated narrations required by the system, eroding credibility and being labelled as an "unreliable witness," and at times as a liar leading to conviction for perjury. The chapter narrates the experience of conducting a workshop on "Testimonies of trauma: Assisting judges understand troubled narratives" at the Delhi Judicial Academy.

As part of a psychoanalytical intervention in judicial training, workshops on "Minimizing the impact of biases, prejudices and stereotypes on the decision making process" were conducted at the Delhi Judicial Academy, Karnataka Judicial Academy and the National Judicial Academy. Sitting on a high dais as a resource person conducting the workshop, the deference and respect shown by the participant judges sitting at a lower level was striking. It immediately brought to mind the almost total reversal of dynamics if I were to be appearing as a lawyer in their court. In turn, it led to the importance placed on setting in therapy. And, perhaps how the setting determines how things appear to us – the view of the factory manager and the worker as to the cause of industrial dispute are a product of the respective locations. The view of an upper-caste person and lower-caste individual may be at polar opposites with regard to slights and humiliations. The workshops attempt to initiate a process of bringing into the conscious the unconscious biases at work opening space for personal introspection and -review. The chapter "Inner World of Judges: Psychoanalytical Explorations" gives an account of the frame of the interventions using the methodology of giving primacy to 'affect' and 'free association' in the training sessions.

The penultimate chapter titled ""Us" and "Them": The Psychology of Inter-community relations" attempts to look beneath the surface at the intra- and inter-psychic processes at play in the raging tensions and conflicts among various communities in India. It examines the application of the formula of picking up a historical trauma acting as if it happened yesterday and conflating the perpetrators at the time with the present targeted community. This reflects a phenomenon that has played out in other parts of the world as well. The bombing of Hiroshima and Nagasaki was preceded by the depiction during World War II of the "enemy" Japanese as subhuman, barbaric, bloodthirsty vermin. Slobodan Milosevic picked up the defeat of Serbia in 1389 and conflated the present-day Bosnian Muslims with Ottoman Turks who were victorious in the Battle of Kosovo, whipping up fury that led to ethnic cleansing in 1995. In India, Lal Krishna Advani, a prominent leader of the Bharatiya Janata Party (BJP), picked up trauma of the destruction of the Somnath Temple in 1025 by Mongols. He then proceeded to deceptively conflate timelines and collapse the identity of the Indian Muslims of today with the invaders. In September 1990, he embarked on a journey from the temple in Gujarat to Babri Masjid in Ayodhya, the birthplace of Rama in the epic Ramayana, whipping up murderous anger leading to riots and killings.

The chapter explores ways to process the trauma of historical events that are selectively mobilized by leaders to target the chosen "enemy" community.

The trauma of partition of India in 1947 remained unacknowledged for a period of 70 years. Invisibilized, it remained festering under the skin impacting events, inter-community relations, courts and inter-religious relationships. The Partition Museum, Amritsar opened in 2017 is the first such attempt at coming to terms with the emotions evoked by the event. The 1954 within a decade of the nuclear attack on 6 August 1945.

The Hiroshima Peace Memorial Museum with artifacts; the Cenotaph for the Atomic Bomb Victims and the Children's Peace Monument are pioneering attempts at processing continuing inter-generational trauma. The Nagasaki Peace Memorial with a Peace Statute and the fountain offers water to the souls of the desperately thirsty victims of the blast.

The Vietnam Veterans War Memorial in Washington D.C. for American lives is another attempt at processing the trauma. The Partition Museum in Amritsar visualized as a Peoples Museum and comprised of people's artifacts and everyday objects is an excellent illustration of initiating processes of acknowledgment and mourning with regard to the trauma of the partition of India into two entities Pakistan and India in 1947. It offers hope as to the possibilities of addressing the sense of grievance and injury of past events that continue to directly impact current socio-political realities in the Subcontinent.

Carrying the thread forward the final chapter titled "Masculinity and Authoritarianism in India" explores links between male sexuality and the characteristic hegemonic hallmark of fascism – the pushing of the singular One Nation, One language, One Leader, One Food, One Religion agenda in India. In each society, there are socio-cultural aspects that enmesh into a totalitarian ideology. The chapter takes the basic premise of Reich that suppression of sexuality leads to a repression in the psyche making an individual subservient, docile and obedient to authority in contrast to material scarcity, which evokes rebellious feelings and explores the specific factors that fed into and led to an exponential growth of the ideology in India. Unlike the Oedipal story, it examines the impact of the myths in India about the son giving up virility for father.[4] The high cultural value placed on celibacy, linking it to spiritual growth as well as the notion of semen as repository of strength and its loss leading to weakness, is dissected to see its role in making the psyche prey to reactionary ideologies preaching hatred against certain designated "enemy" communities. The impact of the revered Mother as Goddess to be worshipped along with unarticulated anxieties evoked by a fearsome, emasculating mother is scrutinized to understand the processes of demonizing the designated "Enemy Community." The splitting of shame evoking feelings like dirtiness and lust and projecting onto the other and in turn, simultaneously stoking anxieties about the rapacious enemy males raping and polluting our pure mothers and sisters, are explored. The devising of collective processes for a community to acknowledge and take back feelings of pollution, dirt and lust is indicated as a possible avenue to explore.

Individual therapy work in the clinic forms the heart of psychoanalysis and the practice of law in courts is the fulcrum of the legal system. The teaching of law and psychology in India is theoretical, with little connection with the practice of law or therapy. An unconscious instinct seems to have driven me to engage with the core of both disciplines. The book is offered as a minor contribution to the increasing trend of psychoanalysis and law to engage with the issues of our times of race, of wars, of xenophobia, of migrations, of refugees, of genocide, of climate change, of breaking out of the binaries of male and female, of internecine violence between communities. Such explorations might offer hope to open up constructive avenues to explore paths towards a more harmonious existence and a more equitable world.

Notes

1 Shukla, R. Of the Bar, the Bench, the Couch, the Flag and Anxious "Love."
2 Please see chapter "Aspects of male sexuality enmeshing with the rise of fascism in India – tentative psychoanalytical explorations."
3 See Shukla, R. https://thewire.in/law/the-perils-of-practising-law-in-a-polarised-environment.
4 As to the father-son myths in India, see chapter "Aspects of male sexuality enmeshing with the rise of fascism in India: Tentative psychoanalytical explorations."

Bibliography

Breuer, J. 1893–1897. Studies in Hysteria. Revised Standard Edition, Vol. II.
Freud, S. 1915. Five lectures on psychoanalysis. Revised Standard Edition, Vol. XI.
Freud, S. 1918. Lines of advance in psychoanalytic therapy. Revised Standard Edition, Vol. XVII.
Freud, S. 1921. Group psychology and the Analysis of the Ego. Revised Standard Edition, Volume XVIII.
Glover, William C. 2023. Psychoanalysis—More than a Profession: Presidential Address, American Psychoanalytic Association, New York, February 3, 2023. https://journals.sagepub.com/doi/pdf/10.1177/00030651241227573 Retrieved 20th February 2026.
hooks, bell. 1984. Feminist Theory from Margin to Centre. South End Press. Boston. https://xyonline.net/sites/xyonline.net/files/2021-12/hooks%2C%20Feminist%20Theory%20-%20From%20Margin%20to%20Center%20%281984%29%20-%20Chap%202%20only.pdf#:~:text=The%20foundation%20of%20future%20feminist%20struggle%20must,underlying%20cultural%20basis%20and%20causes%20of%20sexism. Retrieved 10th March 2026.
hooks, bell. 2000. All About Love: New Visions. William Morrow – an imprint of Harper Collins Publishers. https://dn790000.ca.archive.org/0/items/all-about-love-new-visions-bell/All-About-Love-New-Visions-Bell.pdf#:~:text=There%20can%20be%20no%20love%20without%20justice.,we%20live%20in%20a%20culture%20that%20not&text=Most%20of%20us%20are%20raised%20to%20believe,will%20either%20find%20love%20in%20our%20first. Retrieved 10th March 2026.

Kakar, S. (1989). Intimate relations, exploring Indian sexuality. Penguin Books. New Delhi, India.

Russel, Jacoby. 1983. The Repression of Psychoanalysis, Otto Fenichel and the political Freudians. Basic Books, Inc., Publishers. New York. https://cominsitu.wordpress.com/wp-content/uploads/2021/08/russell-jacoby-the-repression-of-psychoanalysis-1.pdf Retrieved 22 February 2026.

Shukla, R. 2016. Of the Bar, the Bench, the Couch, the Flag and Anxious "Love." Int. J. Appl. Psychoanal. Studies, Vol. 13, No. 2, pp. 185–188 (2016).

Tagirov, Philipp. 2017. The Repressive Hypothesis: Natural Sexuality, Suppressed Eros and a Chance of an Alternative? Advances in Social Science, Education and Humanities Research, volume 124. International Conference on Contemporary Education, Social Sciences and Humanities (ICCESSH 2017). The%20 Repressive%20Hypothesis.pdf. Retrieved 9th March 2026.

1 Gods and Demons
The Murderous Impulses of the Ordinary

At the impressionable age of 13, thanks to a Jesuit priest of Scottish origins whose name has got lost in the mists of time, I was catapulted into the world of William Golding's *Lord of the Flies*. Akin to the idyllic island of the story of *Robinson Crusoe* (Defoe, 1719) which perhaps demonstrates the virtues of hard work, application and faith, it is the story of schoolboys of an elite British school whose plane gets shot down on a tropical island. But Lord of the Flies bears witness to the boys' rapid descent into bloodlust.

> *"Kill the beast! Cut his throat! Spill his blood!"*
>
> ....
>
> *"Kill the beast! Cut his throat! Spill his blood! Do him in!*
>
> ....
>
> *At once the crowd surged after it, poured down the rock, leapt on to the beast, screamed, struck, bit, tore. There were no words, and no movements but the tearing of teeth and claws."*
>
> (pp. 186–187)
>
> *"But really, thought Ralph, this was not Bill. This was a savage whose image refused to blend with that ancient picture of a boy in shorts and shirt."*
>
> (p. 227)
>
> Golding (1954)

The good Jesuit Father also chose as a class reading, "The Crucible" by Arthur Miller written in 1953 about the Salem witch trials in 1692. In retrospect, it seems the display of a rare political acumen in choosing a play pointing to the McCarthyism of the times. A fitting choice to the trilogy was *Macbeth* as the third prescribed book for English Literature. Perhaps, consciously and unconsciously these books led to a lifelong engagement with the ordinariness of murderous impulses, the enmeshing of the individual psyche with group actions and the phenomenon of unconscious guilt.

The poignant cry of Lady Macbeth post-murder of Duncan, "Will all the perfumes of Arabia sweeten this little hand" merge with the image of the death by suicide of Edward Wirth who set up the system of mass killings in

DOI: 10.4324/9781003626794-2

the Auschwitz Gas Chambers. Lifton (1986) writes of Wirth "A man with a strong reputation as a dedicated physician, and described by inmates who could observe him closely as 'kind,' 'conscientious,' 'decent,' 'polite,' and 'honest,' he was the same man who established the camp's system of selections and medicalized killing and supervised the overall process during the two years in which most of the mass murder was accomplished" (p. 384).

Like the cyclical view in Hindu thought, the wheel of time has come full circle with the International Court of Justice finding it plausible that Israel's actions may violate the Genocide Convention[1] and perhaps the events have deeper lessons for us about human nature.

Furies play

The casting of individuals into neat categories of demons and gods perhaps lessens our distress a little when confronting extreme acts of brutality. The brutal rape of a 23-year-old woman in a Delhi bus in December 2012 resulting in her death led to huge protests. The perpetrators were labelled as "psychopaths" who went "berserk." Accounts by women describe the shouting of sexist expletives by the boys' part of the protest, uncontrolled escalation including burning of barricades and simultaneous beatings by the police accompanied by filthy abuse. The actions were far from controlled and the brutality of the police cannot be categorized as the use of limited force by a disciplined body to contain the situation. "Berserk," the word used to describe the perpetrators, denotes out of control with anger or excitement, wild or frenzied. Shukla (2014a) observes, "The accounts about the protests in New Delhi describe escalation, burning of barricades and use phrases like the police went 'berserk' and 'went on a rampage' hitting out at anyone in sight to describe the evening. In a strange turn of events the phrases are similar to those used to describe the conduct of the perpetrators, and we find that the police and protesters too can be prey to feelings from the spectrum of 'berserkers'." The extremes of brutality like inserting an iron rod in the vagina and pulling out the innards give an idea of the fury. However, perhaps the fury has links with the misogyny exhibited in a myriad ways in everyday life.

A college ditty is illustrative. Quite popular among the "ordinary" boys in elite institutions in India and the source of much merriment by endless repetition of the phrases. The lines are striking interlinking the misogyny of the perpetrators and the average joe – the Rajesh, Rakesh and Ramesh destined to take his respectable place in society as a lawyer, doctor or bureaucrat and go as follows:

There was a woman who was never satisfied
So they built her a p….of steel, And attached it to wheel
Round and round went the wheel, in and out went the p….of steel
Till she was split from the …to the …. And the whole fucking thing was full of shit!

Freud famously postulated "castration anxiety" or the fear of the loss of genitals among boys. Klein explored and deepened our understandings about the nature of the anxiety as being at its core a fear of the obliteration of the self which she termed "annihilation anxiety." Freud (1908) writes "Legends and myths testify to the upheaval in the child's emotional life and to the horror which is linked with the castration complex – a complex which is subsequently remembered by consciousness with corresponding reluctance" (p. 189).

Male anxieties at play

Folk tales from different regions of the world seem to indicate, perhaps, universality and the prevalence of the male anxieties across cultures. Gun (2024) refers to Native American, Japanese, African and European tales and interprets them as them as reflecting domestication of female sexuality and deep-seated anxieties about sexuality, gender roles and the balance of power between men and women offers a tale that ends on a different note. Elvin (1949) refers to a number of myths, "For example in a myth from the West coast of Washington the hero meets a woman whose vagina is set with teeth and when he tries to cohabit with her, she bites off his hand."[2]

A Yukaghir tale is about a "pretty young cannibal girl who kills her husbands on the wedding night. Her method is to tire them out and when they fall into an exhausted sleep to kill them.

The hero, warned in time, wears the girl out instead and when she is asleep finds the instruments of death – an awl and a knife – under her pillow. He thrusts the knife into her heart and the awl up her anus crying 'Iron to iron'. The tools meet inside her body and she dies" (p. 246).

Elvin (1949) observes with regard to myths in India:

> We often find the incident, which occurs also in the Indian stories, where the hero is able to break off the teeth of the woman and enjoy normal intercourse with her. The straightforward Vagina Dentata theme is sometimes combined, as in our stories, with symbolical representations of it, and there are the usual variations of the snake in the vagina and the amputated hand.

Elvin (1949) documents the following myth striking in its similarity to the 2012 Delhi Bus Rape incident and the college ditty referred to earlier:

> ASUR
> Pathar, Chhuri Zamindari
> A Rakshasa was in love with a human girl; from their congress was born a daughter who built the town of Dantipur (the Tooth City).[3] She declared that whoever would sleep with her for one night could marry

> her and be the Raja of that place. Many a prince came to visit her, but when they slept with her she cut off their organs with the two teeth in her vagina, and many a prince went home without his penis. At last two friends came, a Raja's son and an Asur boy. The young prince slept with the girl and his penis was cut off. He came out and told his friend. The Asur boy went into his smithy and made an iron penis hollow inside; this he fitted over his own organ. When he went to the girl, he pushed the instrument violently into her vagina; the teeth closed upon it and broke. He pulled them out and threw them down; they stuck in the ground and turned into *kurkutti* (Little tree plant) roots. These roots do not dry all the year round, and our teeth stick in them. They are the roots of a girl's vagina. Then the Asur boy said, 'Mend my friend's penis or I'll kill you'. She mended it and married the Asur. For the prince she got her father's brother's daughter as wife.
>
> (p. 257)

Kakar (1981) speaks of the myth of the capture of Sukra, the evil guru of the demons who had the power to revive slain demons in the womb. "From Siva's third eye there appeared a horrible woman with flowing hair, a great belly, pendulous breasts, thighs like plantain tree trunks, and a mouth like a great cavern. There were teeth and eyes in her womb. Siva said to her, 'Keep the evil guru of the demons in your womb while I kill Jalandhara [the chief of the demon army], and then release him!' She ran after Sukra and grabbed him, stripped him of his clothes and embraced him. She held him fast in her womb, laughed and vanished" (p. 92).

Dreams much like myths and folk tales tell us about the fears and anxieties in the conscious and the unconscious of the human psyche. Elvin's relates that Landtman (1917) noticed a dream among the Kiwai Papuans, which seems illustrative and excerpts the dream:

> The dreamer was asked by a woman to have connection with her, but did not venture to do so, for her vulva was provided with sharp teeth and opened and closed continuously like a mouth. Again and again he tried to muster up courage but shrank back every time. At last the woman got up and attacked him with a piece of wood, and he fled into the water. But he found that he could not swim, and to add to his horror a crocodile came towards him and was about to catch him when he opened his eyes.[4]
>
> (p. 243)

The dream and tales seem as if constructed as exemplars to establish Freud's postulation of castration complex. Freud (1926) writes "His fear that a horse would bite him, can without any forcing, be given the full sense of a fear that the horse would bite off his genitals, would castrate him" (p. 96). Perhaps, it is Klein's deepening and carrying the notion of castration a step further to the anxiety to annihilation, which offers some insight into the furies evoked in the perpetrators. Klein (1946) observes "I hold that anxiety arises from the operation of the Death Instinct within the organism, is felt as fear of annihilation (death) and takes the form of fear of persecution. The fear of the destructive impulse seems to attach itself at once to an object—or rather it is experienced as fear of an uncontrollable overpowering object." Shukla (2014a) notes "In the Indian context powerful imagery of the Mother Goddess Kali, commonly depicted dancing nude with a garland of human skulls, hands gripping various weapons and decapitating encapsulates the male anxiety of castration and annihilation."

Interlinkages

The incident of the insertion of an iron rod in the vagina in the 2012 bus rape incident referred to earlier is not a sole exception. Intermittently, there are reports of similar insertion of foreign objects in the vagina as in the Rohtak Gang rape case (2017)[5] and the 2022 Ghaziabad Gang rape case.[6] Rees (2011), who had researched the cultural and literary history of the vagina, looked upon the traditional stories as of little contemporary relevance. In the piece titled, 'The shocking mythical tales that underlie attitudes to rape in India,' Rees observes, "I'd treated those stories as scraps, merely remnants of an oral tradition which had few echoes in modern culture and which were safely consigned to the archives of misogyny.

But I was wrong – the same stories reverberate in India today, albeit in different words. In one of the first news stories widely reported outside India, a woman was raped and murdered by a group of men on a bus in Delhi in 2012. Since then, images of murdered Indian women have become more and more common – and it's perhaps little surprise given the views of some of the country's politicians."

The Guardian in a 2025 report titled 'Rusted screws, metal spikes and plastic rubbish: the horrific sexual violence used against Tigray's women,' writes about the brutal abuse, gang rape and insertion of objects into their uteruses.

Elvin (1949) writes:

> In human beings also, particularly among those who have an ambivalent attitude to sex -either because they think it is immoral, or have been frustrated in their youth it is not uncommon to find sexual phantasies of an aggressive or violent type: they imagine themselves forcibly penetrating and tearing the vagina, the partner is made to bleed and even killed. In the normal individual this aggressiveness is moderated and even becomes a type of sexual fore-pleasure.
>
> (p. 247)

In the area of heterosexual intercourse, male anxieties about the inability to perform sexual intercourse or feelings of inadequacy of performance are common themes that surface in clinical work. An approaching situation towards sexual intercourse may feel like an impending school examination of a poorly prepared boy with the specter of failure looming large. Then the worst fears come true and the man is not able to perform, reinforcing the fears about inadequacy and the cycle goes on like a running loop. The spectrum from feelings of intrusion, mild irritation and annoyance to fears of being smothered sucked in and swallowed, the self being obliterated, constitute another recurrent theme.

"Pure" evil and "pure" good

The neat binaries of "good and evil" of fairy tales; the "God/s and Satan/Demons of religion"; the "Hero and Villain" of cinema comfort us, reflect our yearning for a simple world and bear exploration.

If anyone can be labelled as the very epitome of evil, it is Dr. Joseph Mengele, Medical Officer at Auschwitz. Referred to as "Dr. Auschwitz," Mengele conducted his diabolical experiments on identical twins in the concentration camp. Mengele carefully provided the sets of twins with special diets and then killed them with lethal injections and thereafter dissected them. Lifton (1986) writes "Mengele himself administered the injections 'without speaking', and 'as though he were performing regular surgery ... without showing any emotion at all'." Mengele also shot a number of prisoners and was reported to have killed at least one woman by pressing his foot on her body. There were additional reports of his having thrown newborn babies directly into crematoria or open fires. In selecting for death or in killing people himself, "the essence of Mengele was flamboyant detachment – one might say disinterestedness – and efficiency" (p. 347).

Yet, Lifton (1986), after a damning list of the atrocities, rejects the casting of Mengele as not a part of the human species and writes "When Hochhuth[7] wrote of his Mengele figure as 'only playing the part of a human being'," he was trying to simplify Nazism by constructing a figure of such pure evil as to no longer belong to the category of human being. Such an exemplar distills and clarifies evil, and we know enough about Mengele to affirm his qualifications for the category. But even Mengele has shown too many familiar facets of human behaviour for one to leave him in that legendary role and, with Hochhuth, "[refrain] from any further effort to plumb [his] human features. *I have made clear my rejection of the legend of pure ahuman evil, clarifying as it may be, in favor of a commitment to probing motivations and behavior*" (p. 380).

Rees (2011) with regard to Rudolph Höss, the Commandant of Auschwitz, observes "During his working days, Höss presided over the murder of more than a million people, but once he came home he lived the life of a solid, middle-class German husband and father." In a similar vein, Bönisch and Wiegrefe (2014) observe "The murderers and their assistants included Catholics and Protestants, the old and the young, people with double doctorates and poorly educated members of the working class. And the percentage of psychopaths was not higher than the average in society as a whole."

In 1961 under the guise of researching learning and punishment, an experiment was carried out where the subjects were to administer shocks ranging from 30 volts to 450 volts to the learners. The subjects included postal clerks, high school teachers, salesmen, engineers and labourers, with education ranging from not having completed elementary school to doctorates. Miligram (1963) reports, "Of the 40 subjects, 26 obeyed the orders of the experimenter to the end, proceeding to punish the victim until they reached the most potent shock available on the shock generator. At that point, the experimenter called a halt to the session. (The maximum shock is labeled 450 volts, and is two steps beyond the designation: Danger: Severe Shock.)" (p. 376).

Quantitatively speaking, 65% of the subjects totally obeyed the order and administered the maximum shock. Milgram (1974) conveys the texture of the dynamics at play: "When he administers 450 volts, he turns to the experimenter and asks, 'Where do we go from here, Professor?' His tone is deferential and expresses his willingness to be a cooperative subject, in contrast to the learner's obstinacy" (p. 46).

The neighbour next door

The casting of the perpetrators of brutal rapes and tortures as not belonging to the same species as the human species is perhaps a comforting simplification of evil. Reality might however be more disturbing. The air hostess in the flat across, the dentist on the floor below or the bank manager who tortures a boy-servant suspecting him of theft are also the "evil villains."

Jagriti Singh, a dentist in a prestigious hospital in New Delhi, the capital of India, installed 20 surveillance cameras all over the house including the bathroom to monitor and control the activities of domestic servants. In November 2013, Singh was arrested for torture using iron rod, sticks, an iron and horns of a dead animal and beating the maid to death.[8] These are not one-off incidents, as in less than a month, there are reports of Vandana Dhir, the senior executive who brutally tortured the Santhal girl in the Vasant Kunj case or Bira Thoibi, the Air India airhostess who locked up her 12-year-old maid in India and departed to Australia. These could be our next-door neighbours, not monsters belonging to another species but "people like us." Dr. Jagriti, a dental surgeon, probably takes great care to lessen the distress and pain of her patients while performing surgery. Edward Wirth, the doctor who set up the mass killings system, was described as "kind" and conscientious by inmates at Auschwitz had a reputation of a dedicated physician.

Control and omnipotence

Perhaps, seeking control reflected in the setting up of 20 surveillance cameras for monitoring the activities and the murderous rage of Dr. Jagriti Singh at some perceived transgression of the norms of behaviour set by her for maids seem to connect with Mengele's fury when encountering any resistance to his diktat. Lifton (1986) tells us "In another, similar case in which a mother did not want to be separated from her thirteen- or fourteen-year-old daughter, and bit and scratched the face of the SS man who tried to force her to her assigned line, Mengele drew his gun and shot both the woman and the child" (p. 343). Perhaps in contrast to the fascism of Hitler and Mussolini, it is what Foucault (1983) terms "the fascism in us all, in our heads and in our everyday behavior" that connects the fury of the neighbour next door to the rage of Mengele.

Explorations at understanding

The explorations are attempts towards understanding of human behaviour in all its dimensions including the violent and the vicious. Winnicott (2005), a pediatrician-psychoanalyst based on engagement with thousands of mother-child pairs speaking of feelings of omnipotence, observes "The mother, at the beginning, by an almost 100 per cent adaptation affords the infant the opportunity for the illusion that her breast is part of the infant. It is, as it were, under the baby's magical control. The same can be said in terms of infant care in general, in the quiet times between excitements. Omnipotence is nearly a fact of experience." (p. 15).

Rodman (2005) speaking of Winnicott's insights observes "He understood that the transition from having all its needs automatically met, in utero, to a capacity to accept the otherness of the external world, the child would have to develop over a long period of time during which the early sense of omnipotence was gradually succeeded by manageable frustrations" (p. xii).

Babies are often described as going blue with anger and the phrase "infantile rage" is indicative perhaps of the lack of the development of the ability in the child to be able to come to terms with the frustrations of external reality and of the independent existence of things and objects which are not in his/her control. Winnicott (1971) then takes us to the ideal processes that go towards equipping the child to deal with the external reality. "This means that the mother (or part of mother) is in a 'to and fro' between being that which the baby has a capacity to find and (alternatively) being herself waiting to be found. If the mother can play this part over a length of time without admitting impediment (so to speak) then the baby has some experience of magical control, that is, experience of that which is called 'omnipotence' in the description of intrapsychic processes (cf. Winnicott, 1962). In the state of confidence that grows up when a mother can do this difficult thing well (not if she is unable to do it), the baby begins to enjoy experiences based on a 'marriage' of the omnipotence of intra-psychic processes with the baby's control of the actual" (p. 63).

At times, the development of the child may not happen along the lines outlined by Winnicott. The baby may not develop the ability to deal with disappointments and frustrations and may not be able to accept the loss of omnipotence. Shukla (2014b) notes "Vital to the development of the ability to cope with anger is introducing small doses of 'optimal frustration', which is enough to create an environment where the child learns the acceptance of limits." The developmental stage of a healthy middle ground between grandiose omnipotence and a realistic feeling of a degree of control in life may not be reached by the baby. The Winnicottian "'marriage' of the omnipotence of intrapsychic processes with the baby's control of the actual" may not take place.

This inability may enmesh with a backlog of dormant unprocessed infantile rage, which erupts like volcanic lava of murderous fury seen in Mengele and Singh, propelling to torture and killings triggered by perceived departures from the pre-written script of the protagonist. The totally different settings of – a concentration camp and a public hospital; of gender – a male and a female and the time period – Germany of the 1940s and India of the 2010s, and yet a similarity of furies, tend to corroborate with the universality of the intra- and interpsychic processes at play. Winnicott (1971) writes "It is hoped that psychoanalysts will be able to use the theory of transitional phenomena in order to describe the way in which good-enough environmental provision at the very earliest stages makes it possible for the individual to cope with *the immense shock of loss of omnipotence*" (p. 95) (emphasis added).

Perhaps, "the shock of loss of omnipotence" at times remains a continuing sore thread in life. The installing of surveillance cameras by Dr. Jagriti to monitor domestic maids could be an attempt at regaining a sense of omnipotence and power. At other times, the loss of omnipotence perhaps becomes intolerable, exploding with murderous fury when "her" maids deviate from the behaviour laid down for them by Dr. Jagriti. The non-obedience to be in the assigned line as the mother did not want to be separated from her 13-year-old daughter at Auschwitz, triggering rage in Mengele who shoots them dead and sends all the people from that transport to the gas chamber is perhaps an attempt at regaining the lost magical feeling as an infant for whom omnipotence was an experienced "fact."

In the absence of the Winnicottian balance between "omnipotence" and the limited "control of the actual," the self may swing from being the

"Greatest" to being "Nothing," from being the "Hero" of the film to being an insignificant "Extra" in a crowd scene; from the "Most Loved" to "Nobody loved." Shukla (2014b) writes "The other side of this grandiose omnipotent controlling self are feelings of emptiness, worthlessness and being out of control. The individual oscillates between these two extremes" (p. 362).

A person may have inner feelings of being out of control, which may manifest in keeping a strict control of the outside like keeping the desk exactly so with the pen, pencils and erasers in their designated spots, which may be reassuring to the self. On the other hand, an inner feeling of being out of control may be reflected in the outside and keeping things scattered and messy on the desk. The same messy and out-of-control inner feelings may lurk behind the swings between diametrically opposite manifest behaviours of absolute control and a feeling of total lack of control. Perhaps, in the case of individuals like Dr. Jagriti and Mengele, hidden behind the manifest attempt at absolute control over the outside and the fury triggered at the perceived transgression, may lie feelings of impotence and insignificance.

In fact, Lifton (1986) based on extensive interviews of the Auschwitz doctors and survivors observes with regard to the camp personnel, "The Auschwitz self wavered between the sense of omnipotent control over the lives and deaths of prisoners and the seemingly opposite sense of impotence, of being a powerless cog in a vast machine controlled by unseen others … The polarity took on grotesque dimensions in Auschwitz, as Nazi doctors called forth feelings of omnipotence and related sadism on the one hand, and of impotence and sometimes masochism on the other, in order to quiet this death anxiety" (pp. 447–448).

"Honour" killings

In a 2025 video that went viral, a young woman Aanchal Mamidwar is seen kneeling behind the lifeless body of her partner Saksham Tate, smearing *haldi* (turmeric) across his cheeks, *kumkum* (vermilion) to his forehead through uncontrollable sobs, an attempt to fulfil the wedding ceremony they had planned. A day earlier, Saksham had been shot in an autorickshaw, dragged out and bludgeoned to death by her father and brothers because he was from a lower caste. The front-page headline reads "I married my BF's body because I didn't want my family to win."[9]

The case of the killing of Ved Pal who had gone to fetch his wife Sonia armed with a High Court order and accompanied by a court official and policemen speaks volumes of the murderous furies aroused at an individual and a collective level at transgressing rules and deviating from the strict control of the khap or caste panchayat. The khap issued a diktat against marrying in the same *gotra* and sentenced the couple to death for getting married.[10] Gotras are predicated on the belief that all Hindus having descended from certain sages like Bharadwaja, Vashisht, Vishwamitra and so on. The belief that persons from the same gotra are close kin and should not marry has no rational basis, yet frequently the couple is killed for the violation of the diktat. In the case of Ved Pal, a mob gathered, the policemen and court official fled, possibly sharing the beliefs of the khap-caste panchayat. Shukla (2010) explores the processes at play in "Honor" Killings: A Look Within the Psyche. Ved Pal was dragged out of the room where he had taken shelter and beaten to death reported as "Youth beaten to death for marrying."

A village in rural India and a concentration camp; local khap-caste panchayat and the Head Doctor Auschwitz, the settings could not be more divergent, yet the sentencing to death and the brutal beating of Ved Pal for transgression of the *khap*-caste *panchayat* rule may be a pointer to the universality of intra- and interpsychic processes at play in the human mind. Lifton (1986) notes, "For Mengele's studied detachment could be interrupted by outbreaks of rage and violence, especially when encountering resistance to his sense of the Auschwitz rules … … [Mengele then] grabbed me by the hair, dragged me on the ground, and beat me. When my mother also tried to beg him, he beat her with his cane [riding crop]" (p. 343). Dr. Jagriti used iron rod, sticks, an iron and horns of an animal and beat the maid to death somewhat akin to the riding crop of Mengele.

Public lynching

The cow is revered as Mother by a sizable section of upper-caste Hindus. Such is also the case in the village of Bisada, on the outskirts of India's capital, Delhi. An announcement by the priest from a temple in the village, that beef was being eaten in the house of the victim, evokes anger in the predominant community of the upper-caste Thakurs in the village is in the realm of the comprehensible. However, the explosion of murderous fury leading to the lynching of Aqlakh and the beating to near death of the son Danish in September 2015 is indicative of deep currents running under the surface. The fact that Danish is a serving Indian Air Force officer whose patriotism could not be questioned does not seem to have deterred the group from almost killing him. Unlike, the anonymity of a big city, the mob which lynched Aqlakh were his neighbours' and fellow-residents who had lived all their life in the village together and knew each other well.

Even the idea of slaughtering a cow (which was not borne out by evidence) igniting such intense fury propelling the group to kill an elderly Muslim gentleman who probably they saw on way to school in their childhood demands a deeper look at the dynamics at play.

Psychoanalytical explorations killing of Akhlaq

The killing of a Hindu mother triggering a murderous fury leading to killing Akhlaq would fall within the framework of retribution as justice. There were no possibilities of sessions with the accused perpetrators in the killing as a psychoanalyst, towards an attempt to unpack the conundrum of the rumour of the killing of a cow igniting rage of an intensity leading to the beating of another human being, a helpless elderly Muslim gentleman to death. "Shukla (2016) in "Beef, Murderous Rage, Public Lynching: A Look under the Surface" attempts to explore the dynamics." In a curious turn of events, Mohammed Ali, a journalist who extensively covered the Akhlaq killing for a national daily, contacted me for therapy. The experience provided a unique entry point and window into the events. Ali wanted to be named and graciously gave consent to the following paragraph.

Interviewing the perpetrators – The memories of Mohammed Ali

As part of professional duties as a journalist, Mohammed Ali had to cover the killing of Akhlaq. The work involved extensive meetings and interviews with the persons accused of the murder of Akhlaq. Like Akhlaq, Ali is a Muslim and the accused were Hindus. This involved fraternizing with the accused, including having tea with them, laughing along with at anti-Muslim jokes and listening to their tirades. The Hindu accused of course knew that Ali was a Muslim and perhaps, in some species of the exercise of heady majoritarian power made a point of voicing their prejudices about Muslims in his presence. The gamut of emotions the experience of these interactions evoked brought B to the doors of my clinic.

Ali (2021) speaking of his experience of interviewing the perpetrators writes, "Lying on the therapist's brown couch, next to a tissue box, I find myself returning to a dark memory. I am in an unfamiliar drawing room, sipping tea, my reporter's notebook on the table before me. … What he does know is my Muslim name, just a word removed from Mohammed Akhlaq, the fifty-two year old man he and a mob of Hindu vigilantes lynched a few months earlier, on the night of September 28, 2015, less than fifty meters from where we are sitting. Several of his associates surround him as I try to strike up a conversation. …

My body breaks into a sweat, despite the December cold. As S. rants about the villainies of Islam, I stay guarded, tight-lipped, keeping speech to a minimum, asking for a clarification here and a detail there, steering clear of any sentiments that might reveal my Muslim-ness, betray my helplessness. Soon, I feel a sense of guilt welling up. A terrible thought crosses my mind: Am I colluding with him, sitting here in his house, without protesting? .... As I leave his house, I imagine S. laughing behind my back, taunting me, dismissing me as a deluded reporter and a *katua*—an Islamophobic slur reducing Muslim men to their circumcised penis—on top of that.... No matter how critical I am about their actions, I fear I am, at the end of the day, enabling the violent ideology of Hindutva by 'humanizing' its followers, not to mention providing the media attention they crave."

The setting, the events, the circumstances and the dramatis personae are decades apart, yet we find that the emotions Lifton, who belonged to the Jewish faith and had extensive interviews with the doctors of Auschwitz, articulates strike a chord with Ali's, "Yet it was in those sitting rooms that I did a great part of the research, and did it in a way that required me to view medical perpetrators, what- ever their relationship to evil, as human beings and nothing else. That meant requiring of myself a form of empathy for Nazi doctors: I had to imagine my way into their situation, not to exonerate but to seek knowledge of human susceptibility to evil... Yet whatever its logic, it felt strange and uncomfortable to hold out even minimal empathy (and even with full awareness of the clear distinction between empathy and sympathy) for participants in a project so murderous, and *one aimed specifically at my own people, at me...* One sometimes enters into another's situation not to help but to expose and evaluate motivations and behavior. Even then, one is making human contact, avoiding what Erik Erison has called 'pseudospeciation', or seeing other human beings as belonging to a different species" (pp. 501–502).

Ali's and Lifton's feeling despite their writing frame in which the perpetrators come across as bad and vicious, that interviewing a person means connecting to the individual as a human being. Even after Ali (2020) writing in-depth on Vivek Premi – an anti-Muslim mobilizer and perpetrator of violence was published, the individual connected and received Ali with warmth and felt that he had been presented as a species of human being.[11]

The destructive impulses of the infant

The mother-son bond is revered in Indian society as the purest and most selfless, bordering on the divine, and leaving no room for ambivalence. In tune with this ethos at a manifest level, there are no feelings of antagonism, aggression and resentments experienced by the son towards the mother. The perpetrators of the killing of Akhlaq are all young, upper-caste Hindu men. Our explorations to tease apart the impulses at play take us to the childhood of young boys in general and boys in Hindu families in particular.

Klein (1946) in the context of mother-and-child dynamics at play observes "From the beginning the destructive impulse is turned against the object and is first expressed in phantasised oral-sadistic attacks on the mother's breast which soon develop into onslaughts on her body by all sadistic means. The persecutory fears arising from the infant's oral-sadistic impulses to rob the mother's body of its good contents, and the anal-sadistic impulses to put his excrements into her (including the desire to enter her body in order to control her from within), are of great importance for the development of paranoia and schizophrenia" (p. 99).

Freud (1931) notes that he has not been able to see through any case completely and that women analysts have been more successful in grasping these processes, "It does indeed appear that women analysts – as, for instance Laml-de Groot and Helene Deutsch – have been able to perceive these facts more easily and clearly because they were helped in dealing with those under their treatment by the transference to a suitable mother substitute. Nor have I succeeded in seeing my way through any case completely, and I shall therefore confine myself to reporting the most general findings and give only a few ideas which I have arrived at" (pp. 216–217). After admitting that woman analysts have been able to grasp the processes better, and Klein used the gender-neutral "infant," Freud confines the oral-sadistic impulses towards the mother to the girl-child: "Among these is a suspicion that this phase of attachment to the mother is especially intimately related to the aetiology of hysteria, which is not surprising when we reflect that both the phase and the neurosis are characteristically feminine, and further, that in this dependence on the mother we have the germ of later paranoia in women. For this germ appears to be the surprising but regular fear, of being killed (?) devoured by the mother. It is plausible to assume that this fear corresponds to a hostility which develops in the child towards her mother in consequence of the manifold restrictions imposed by the latter in the course of training and bodily care and that the mechanism of projection is favoured by the early age of the child's psychical organisation" (p. 217). Freud elaborates – "We find the little girl's aggressive oral and sadistic wishes in a form forced on them by early repression, as a fear of being killed by her mother – a fear which in turn, justifies her death-wish against her mother, if that becomes conscious. It is impossible to say how often this fear of the mother is supported by an unconscious hostility on the mother's part which is sensed by the girl" (p. 226).

It is difficult to fathom Freud's confining solely to the girl child the hostility and projection towards the mother. The reason given that it "in consequence of the manifold restrictions imposed by the latter in the course of training and bodily care" is equally applicable to the boy-child. The oral-sadistic and anal-sadistic impulses of the infant are as much at play in the boy. In fact, Freud's postulating that the boy has not only affection, but also jealousy and hostility towards the mother supports the view that the processes operate in both the sexes. Freud (1923) notes – "Closer study usually discloses the *more complete* Oedipus complex, which is two-fold, positive and negative, and is due to the bisexuality present in children: that is to say, a boy has not merely an ambivalent attitude towards his father and an affectionate object choice towards his mother, but at the same time also behaves like a girl and displays an affectionate attitude to his father and a corresponding *jealousy and hostility towards his mother*" (emphasis added). This finds further support from Freud's (1931) observations: "(Hitherto, it is only in men that I have found the fear of being eaten up. This fear is referred to the Father, but it is probably the product of the transformation of oral aggressivity directed to the mother. The child wants to eat up its mother from whom it has had its nourishment; in the case of the father there is no such obvious determinant of the wish)" (p. 226).

In fact, Freud (1909) reports the following session with "Little Hans":

> 'I: "Would you like to beat Mummy, Hanna or me?"
> 'Hans: "Mummy."
> 'I: "Why?"
> 'Hans: "I should just like to beat her."
>
> (p. 62)

Little Hans' desire to beat up his mother indicating aggression meshes in with a possible thread of the unconscious hostility of the perpetrators towards their respective mothers and consequent guilt, evoking murderous fury leading to the beating to death of Akhlaq, the perceived killer of the mother-cow.

Of boy-gods and mothers

The story of the creation of the elephant-headed Ganesha is instructive in an exploration of the mother-son bond in India. There are invariably several versions of any of the prevalent myths. A summary of one version is as follows: Parvati, the consort of the God Shiva, wanted to bathe and wanted someone to guard against intrusion. Parvati formed the figurine of a boy from the dirt and the turmeric cleansing paste of her body and breathed life in it. Shiva returned and wanted to enter and was stopped by Ganesha who was unaware that Shiva was his father. A furious Shiva beheaded the boy. An enraged Parvati threatened to destroy the entire creation. Shiva brought the head of an elephant, the first living creature he encountered and attached it to the body of the boy, thus creating the elephant-headed boy God.

The creation of the figurine of the boy from the dirt of the body of the mother without the participation of the father is striking in the total fusion of the mother and the boy-child. The exclusive loyalty of the child to the mother to the exclusion of the father shapes the psyche of the growing boy in a Hindu family even in the present times. The mother-son bond gets compounded by marital tensions between husband and wife. Ganesha is depicted as a permanently chubby asexual boy-child who cannot be imagined with sexual desires and wishes and the purpose of whose creation is the service and comfort of the mother. These tropes are manifested in everyday practices. In the prevalent traditional practice of arranged marriage, the son seeks a wife who will see to the comfort and happiness of the mother. In the context of Shiva beheading Ganesha, Ramanujam (1999) in the paper "The Indian Oedipus" refers to a number of myths in India, which end up with the son giving up virility and potency.[12]

Clinical material emerging in the course of more than a decade and a half of practice consistently shows that it is fairly common practice to continue the breast feeding of the male offspring till the age of 4–5 and at times even 8–9 years in India. Often, the longing for a son translates into the male offspring, being the youngest sibling preceded by three to four sisters. So the stopping and tapering of breastfeeding on the birth of a younger sibling does not occur. Even if there is no milk in the breast of the mother to feed the child, yet the mother puts the breast to the mouth of the child. At times, there is a stray remark or two by relatives or neighbours that the child is perhaps a bit old to be breastfed. This is promptly responded to by the mother as a demand of the child-son. Indulgence of a desired for precious son after three daughters is something everyone understands. Any parent with three daughters has sympathy in society as it needs no explanation that they are byproducts on the way to have a male offspring.

The mother may consciously think of and couch it in terms of the son's need and demand, but at an unconscious level, it may perhaps be the longing and wish of the mother for closer sensuous proximity and connectedness. At times, the son may be feeling overwhelmed, smothered and suffocated by the breasts, yet the setting has no space to deviate from the paradigm of the "fond mother indulging the demanding son" by giving her breasts to him. At a conscious level, the son accepts the paradigm and does not have the wherewithal to articulate the emotions experienced.

Kakar (1981) notes "Setting aside our consideration of the unconscious for a moment, we can observe that an Indian child tends to experience his mother almost totally as a 'good mother'" (p. 83). Elaborating on the theme, Kakar observes "For a range of reasons, the balance of nurturing may be so affected that the mother unconsciously demands that the child serve as an object of her own unfulfilled desires and wishes, however antithetical they may be to his own. The child feels compelled then to act as her saviour. Faced with her unconscious intimations and demands, he may feel confused, helpless and inadequate, frightened by his mother's overwhelming nearness and yet unable (and partly unwilling) to get away" (p. 89).

In sharp contrast to Western practice of separate bedrooms for parents and children, it is fairly prevalent for children to be sleeping with their parents in the same bed till a relatively late age. Clinical work consistently shows that at times, the boy-child witnesses sexual intercourse in a half-asleep state or while pretending to sleep and gets aroused and excited. This in turn may bring intolerable intense feelings of guilt at the lust experienced for the 'sacred' mother.

At times, the son may experience longings to take the mother's place, with the father again evoking acute guilt. This can open up a Pandora's Box of emotions – ranging from feelings of inadequacy, anxieties as to performance, of being subsumed or devoured and may put brakes on or at times lead to a cessation of desire.

Small canvas camping tents by the side are a common sight on highways and roads in India. These are temporary shifting residence-cum-clinics of the traditional healers of the Unani and Ayurvedic systems of medicine. They primarily cater to male anxieties around sexual performance, which seems to be the major source of income. Shukla (2015) notes "Psychoanalytical insights apart the insecurities of the Indian male pertaining to sex are succinctly put down and encashed by sundry traditional healers in posters in public toilets across the country offering solutions to sexual problems of males by traditional healers" (see text for details). The accompanying poster stuck on a public toilet wall in Delhi representative of the genre titled "Sex Power+Obstacle" roughly translated lists them as Looseness in sex; Small/Crooked/Thin penis; Sins of childhood (euphemistic reference to masturbation) and Low sperm count. Transgender sex workers are often at the receiving end of violence by male clients. Perhaps at an unconscious level, male insecurities of "not being man enough" get triggered in the male clients. Shukla (2013) notes, "The transgender 'hijra' and 'kothi' do not fit into the neat binary of 'man' and 'woman' and seem to invite particularly vicious violations of a sexual nature by local *goondas* and hoodlums in the place of business, usually public parks" (p. 230).

In sync with myths about vagina dentita reported by Gun, G. (2024) and annihilation anxieties, Kakar (1981) observes that the vagina can be perceived as "the entrance into the depths of a death womb which takes life back into itself" (p. 89). Kakar takes the thread forward, pointing to male fears of performance, "One of the likely psycho-sexual consequences of this anxiety provoking process of association in unconscious fantasy is a heightened fear, or the actual occurrence, of impotence" (p. 95). This seamlessly meshes in with the popularity of traditional healers whose main business is the treatment of male anxieties about lack of potency.

Devotion and rage

At a conscious and social level, there is no acknowledgement of any feelings of aggression or hostility in the pure spiritual and sacred mother-son bond. It is likely that at an individual level, the aggressive feelings towards the mother are too intolerable for the boy-child, and instead are suppressed and transformed into fear of the marauding – decapitating-devouring Mother. In turn at a collective level, it may be reflected in the fearsome image of the Mother-Goddess Kali blood dripping with a severed head in hand, a garland of skulls around the neck with tongue sticking out found in grand temples as well as non-descript roadside shrines.

The rage at mother could not in a linear way be directly projected at a Muslim mother as it is still too proximate and unbearable. Perhaps, the rage at the loving and revered mother required a further distancing before the split-off anger could surface in the step of displacement to the cow-mother. The absolute suppression and lack of acknowledgement of even the possibility of anger towards the mother perhaps surfaced as unconscious part-identification with the killer of the cow. Thus, the belief that a cow had been killed on the one hand may have triggered rage at the taking away of the nourishing milk-giving breast and simultaneously led to splitting, projection and projective identification. The splitting of suppressed and splitoff unacknowledged and unarticulated resentments, hostility and fears about the mother; the splitoff parts get projected onto the Muslim men Akhlaq and his son and the third step part-identification with the Muslim men who killed the mother-cow. The feelings of virulent anger evoked by unconscious part-identification with the killers of the mother-cow may have synergistically meshed in with the rage triggered at the taking away of the nourishing milk-giving cow propelling the murderous fury and the beating to death of Akhlaq. The women in the house seem to have not been attacked, perhaps corroborating the hypothesis of projective identification with the men perceived as killers of the cow.

Remorse and reparation <> Ahuman and incorrigible

> Choice, however, is a vexing word. What part of choice applies when a tidal wave of anger tears through a state? What part of it is the moment, the madness, the collective, and what part individual, personal history?
>
> Laul (Front cover flap)

The issue of sole individual responsibility for a crime and the role of the social factors in the nature of poverty, systemic humiliations, dysfunctional family, childhood trauma, intergenerational trauma of a marginalized community being contributing factors come to the fore starkly in the context of the imposition of death penalty on an individual. The juvenile accused in the 2012 Delhi Bus Gang rape case (2012) came from a poor family in a village in Uttar Pradesh and migrated to Delhi at the tender age of 11. He did various menial jobs like working in roadside eateries where he would have got regularly beaten up and assaulted.

The systematic killings of Muslims in 2002 in the Gujarat state of India mark a turning point in the history of India and have been extensively documented by rights groups.[13] In sharp contrast to the torture, rape and killing by official instrumentalities of the state to be lured by your trusted neighbour with promise of protection and then locked up in a room and killed perhaps breaks human trust at a qualitatively different level.

Laul (2018), author of the book "The Anatomy of Hate," met approximately a hundred people who participated in the killings and conducted extensive interviews with three of them. Suresh Jadeja alias Suresh Langdo participated in one of the worst killings in Naroda Patiya, a neighbourhood in the city of Ahmedabad and in the murder of a full-term Muslim Kauser-bi – ripping the foetus out with a sword, and seems the personification of Evil Incarnate. Laul writes about his childhood "For Suresh growing up was like light going out of his eyes .... Polio gave Suresh his middle name as a child, one everyone in Charranagar used: Langdo, the limper" (p. 36). Laul recounts the testimony of a man who has seen Suresh since he was ten years old. "Suresh and my son got into a scuffle, he hit my son and stole his watch. I registered a complaint with the local police," he said. "And the cops came after Suresh and beat the crap out of him. They went on beating him over and over again." (p. 38). The unprocessed feelings of helplessness, rage and impotence evoked by experiences growing up as a child perhaps burst in volcanic fury in the setting of a mob on the rampage against Muslims.

Lifton (1986) observes "Under certain conditions, just about anyone can join a collective call to eliminate every last one of the alleged group of carriers of the 'germ of death'" (p. 503). The second and third protagonists of Laul are remorseful. Dungar, who led the burning of Muslim houses in a reparative gesture, helps in rebuilding the houses. Pranav who accompanied his hostel mates and friends in looting and burning of Muslim shops was deeply impacted by visits to the refugee camps, and got involved in efforts at building bridges between the communities through joint cricket teams of Hindus and Muslims.

It is the categorization of an individual as beyond regret, remorse and reform and having no redeeming qualities, which has been the basis of capital punishment. The bedrock of executing people is the hypothesis of the "Born Incorrigible Criminal" pioneered in criminal jurisprudence by

Lombroso (1876).[14] This brings us back to the circular logic of the demonization at a collective level of certain communities as subhuman by the perpetrators. And in turn categorizing the perpetrators as Lifton (1986) puts it as "pure ahuman evil."

Journalist Nidhi Suresh (2025) interviewed rape accused Pulsar Suni, over a period of 13 months. Suni was convicted on 8 December 2025 for the abduction and rape of a leading Malayalam actor. Suresh observes, "As a journalist, I had trained myself to be interested in the grey, to be cautious of neat stories and suspicious of linear narratives. But this was a frightening shade for grey — It was not his extraordinary capability for violence, but the stunning ordinariness with which he met people."

We can do no better than agree with Lifton as he succinctly differentiates taking on board murderous impulses from acting them out, "One of these distinctions concerns how, with our universal potential for murder and genocide, we for the most part hold back from such evil" (p. 503).

Acknowledging that each of us is capable of killing perhaps places even more of an existential responsibility for our actions. It is the human facets and in a sense the ordinariness of the perpetrators which are scary and despairing, but perhaps also a pointer and source of hope and redemption.

Notes

1 South Africa versus Israel (2024). International Court of Justice. Order 26 January 2024.
2 Goddard, Jicarilla Apache Texts, 202 f.
3 Dantewada – literally meaning the place of residence of the tooth – is very much a real town in Bastar region of Chhatisgarh, India, which the author has had occasion to visit.
4 Landtman, Folk Tales, No. 398.
5 Rohtak Gang rape case: Skull shattered, sharp objects inserted into private parts, reveals investigation.
6 "Woman gang-raped, rod inserted; condition critical." Jhelum Times, Uttar Pradesh, 19 October 2022.
7 Refers to the creation by Rolph Hochhuth of a Mengele-like character known as "the doctor" as Absolute Evil in the play *The Deputy*.
8 This was reported as "Domestic help beaten to death, BSP MP, wife arrested". Hindustan Times, by HT Correspondent, New Delhi. Updated 6 November 2013, 2:19 p.m. IST.
9 I married my BF's body because I didn't want my family to win." Times of India. Bengaluru. 8 December 2025.
10 Youth beaten to death for marrying. https://www.ndtv.com/india-news/youth-beaten-to-death-for-marrying-398516. Retrieved 8 December 2025.
11 The Rise of a Hindu Vigilante in the Age of WhatsApp and Modi. Mohammed Ali.

12 See Chapter 7 – Masculinity and Authoritarianism in India.
13 Harvest of Hatred—The Concerned Citizens' Report on Gujarat, 2002, Manohar books; "Maro! Kaapo! Balo!" – State, Society and Communalism in Gujarat, Peoples' Union for Democratic Rights (PUDR), May 2002; "We Have No Orders to Save You" – State Participation and Complicity in Communal Violence in Gujarat, April 2002, Human Rights Watch April 2002 Vol. 14, No. 3 (C).
14 Criminal Man. Cesare Lombroso. 1856.

Bibliography

Ali, Mohammed. 2020. The rise of a Hindu vigilante in the age of WhatsApp and Modi. Wired. https://www.wired.com/story/indias-frightening-descent-social-media-terror/. Retrieved 5th February 2026.

Ali, Mohammed. 2021. The Scream – Is this the end for Muslims in India. The baffler. https://thebaffler.com/salvos/the-scream-ali. Retrieved 5th February 2026.

Bönisch, G., & Wiegrefe, K. 2014. Spiegel online international. http://www.spiegel.de/international/germany/everyday-murder-nazi-atrocities-committed-byordinary-people-a-542245.html. Retrieved 6th August 2014.

camus-neither-victims-nor-executioners.pdf Retrieved 2nd December 2025.

Defoe, Daniel. 1719. Robinson Crusoe. Willaim Taylor. Great Britain.

Domestic help beaten to death, BSP MP, wife arrested. https://www.hindustantimes.com/india/domestic-help-beaten-to-death-bsp-mp-wife-arrested/story-IDD33sabpy8yUaV1Cd3uBN.html. Retrieved 7th December 2025.

Elvin, Verrier. 1949. Myths of middle India. First Published in 1949 by Geoffrey Cumberlege, Oxford University Press. Madras. https://www.arvindguptatoys.com/arvindgupta/myths-verrier.pdf. Retrieved 3rd February 2026

Foucault, M. (1983). Preface. In Anti-Oedipus. University of Minnesota Press. Deleuze & Guaattari Minneapolis, MN.

Freud, S. 1908. 'Civilized' sexual morality and modern nervous illness. Revised Standard Edition Volume IX.

Freud, S. 1909. Analysis of a phobia in a five-year-old boy. Revised Standard Edition Vol. X.

Freud, S. 1923. The ego and the id. Revised Standard Edition IX.

Freud, S. 1926(1925). Inhibitions, symptoms and anxiety. Revised Standard Edition Vol. XX.

Freud, S. 1931. Female sexuality. Revised Standard Edition XXI.

Golding, W. 1954. Lord of the flies. https://lexiconic.net/english/LordoftheFlies.pdf Retrieved 5th December 2025.

Gun, Gary. 2024. Exploring the vagina dentata myth: A cultural analysis. https://socialattraction.co.uk/exploring-the-vagina-dentata-myth-a-cultural-analysis/ Retrieved 6th December 2025.

Harvest of Hatred—The Concerned Citizens' Report on Gujarat, 2002, Manohar books; "Maro! Kaapo! Balo!" – State, Society and Communalism in Gujarat, Peoples' Union for Democratic Rights (PUDR), May 2002; "We Have No Orders to Save You" – State Participation and Complicity in Communal Violence in Gujarat, April 2002, Human Rights Watch April 2002 Vol. 14, No.3(C).

Kakar, S. 1981. The Inner World, A Psychoanalytic Study of Childhood and Society in India. Oxford University Press. Delhi.

Landtman, Gunnar. 1917. The folk-tales of the Kiwai Papuans. Helsingfors: Print. Office of the Finnish Society of Literature, 1917.

Lifton, Robert J. 1986. The Nazi Doctors - Medical Killing and the Psychology of Genocide. Basic Books Inc. New York. Retrieved 2nd December 2025

Lombroso, Cessare. 1876. L'uomo inquente. Publisher Ulrico Hoepli. MiCriminal Man, According to the Classification of Cesare Lombroso. 1911. G.P. Putnam's Sons. New York.

Klein, M. 1946. Notes on some schizoid mechanisms. International Journal of Psychoanalysis, Vol. 27, pp. 99–110. https://dravni.co.il/wp-content/uploads/2015/11/Klein-M.-1946.-Notes-on-Some-Schizoid-Mechanisms.pdf

Laul, R. 2018. The Anatomy of Hate. Context, an imprint of Westland Publications. Chennai, India.

Miligram, Stanley. 1963. Behavioural Study of Obedience. Journal of Abnormal and Social Psychology, Vol. 67, No. 4, pp. 371. https://www.columbia.edu/cu/psychology/terrace/w1001/readings/milgram.pdf. Retrieved 11th February 2026.

Milgram, Stanley. 1974. Obedience to Authority, An Experimental View. Tavistock Publications Ltd. London. https://www.psicopolis.com/psicopedia/boxpdf/milgram2.pdf. Retrieved 11th February 2026.

Ramanujam, A. K. 1999. The Indian Oedipus. In T. G. Vaidyanthan & J. J. Kirpal (Eds.), Vishnu on Freud's Desk. OUP. Delhi, India.

Rees, L. 2011. Rudoph Höss– Commandant of Auschwitz. http://www.bbc.co.uk/history/worldwars/genocide/hoss_commandant_auschwitz_01.shtml. Retrieved 6th August 2014.

Rodman. F. Robert. 2005. Preface. Playing and Reality. Winnicott. D.W. Routledge Classics 2005. Routledge. Abingdon, Oxon.

Rohtak Gang rape case: Skull shattered, sharp objects inserted into private parts, reveals investigation. May 14, 2017. https://www.india.com/news/india/rohtak-gang-rape-case-skull-shattered-sharp-objects-inserted-into-private-parts-reveals-investigation-2132413/ Retrieved 4th February 2026.

Landtman, Gunnar. 1917. The Folk-Tales of the Kiwai Papuans. Print. Office of the Finnish Society of Literature. Helsingfors.

Shukla, R. 2010. "Honor" Killings: A Look Within the Psyche. The International Journal of Applied Psychoanalytic Studies, Vol. 7, No. 1, pp. 85–87.

Shukla, R. 2013. A walk through the labyrinths of sex work law in Murthy, Laxmi and Seshu. In Meena Saraswathi (Ed.), The Business of Sex. Zubaan. Delhi.

Shukla, R. 2014a. The Rage of Angels: Anger, Fury, Brutal Rape, Protests, Police Action. The International Journal of Applied Psychoanalytic Studies, Vol. 11, No. 2, pp. 184–187.

Shukla, R. 2014b. The Murderous Rage of the Ordinary: A Perspective from India. The International Journal of Applied Psychoanalytic Studies, Vol. 11, No. 4, pp. 360–362.

Shukla, R. 2015. Sex Workers: Repositories of the "Bad". The International Journal of Applied Psychoanalytic Studies. Vol. 12, No. 2, pp. 181–185.

Shukla, R. 2016. Beef, Murderous Rage, Public Lynching: A Look under the Surface. The International Journal of Applied Psychoanalytic Studies. Published online in Wiley Online Library (wileyonlinelibrary.com). DOI: 10.1002/aps.1489

South Africa versus Israel. Report of the International Court of Justice. Order 26th January 2024. https://www.icj-cij.org/node/203447. Retrieved 2nd February 2026.

Suresh, N. 2025. Inside the Twisted Mind of a Hired Rapist. https://www.thenewsminute.com/premium/inside-the-twisted-mind-of-a-hired-rapist? Retrieved 13th December 2025.

Times of India. Bengaluru. 8th December 2025. "I married my BF's body because I didn't want my family to win".

Woman gang-raped, rod inserted; condition critical. 19 October 2017. Jehlam Times. https://www.facebook.com/JehlamTimes/posts/woman-gang-raped-rod-inserted-condition-crithttradicaluttar-pradesh-the-delhi-commissi/5520149641400336/. Retrieved 4th February 2026.

Winnicott. D.W. 2005. Playing and Reality. Routledge Winnicott Classics. Routledge. Abingdon, Oxon.

Winnicott. D.W. Ego Integration in Child Development. In The Maturational Processes and the Facilitating Environment. London: Hogarth Press and the Institute of Psycho-Analysis, 1965.

Youth beaten to death for marrying. https://www.ndtv.com/india-news/youth-beaten-to-death-for-marrying-398516. Retrieved 8th December 2025.

2 Love and Rage in Intimate Relations: Sorties in Narcissism and Projection

The *"Battle of the Sexes"* appears to be most popularly associated with the internationally televised match between Billie Jean King and Bobby Riggs in 1973, incidentally won by King in three sets. The theme of friction between men and women is a running thread from oral traditions from the 7th Century, the poetry of Wesley, the writings of Freud to the film *Battle of the Sexes* (2017).

Freud's views about women's hostile bitterness in the context of relations between the sexes seem to echo the tales orally narrated through the generations in India. One of the first publications dated to 12 CE is the *Shuka Saptapti* or "Seventy Tales of the Parrot" in Sanskrit. The tales with gnomic stanzas and verses created over centuries have a number of variations and additions from various other texts. Many are direct and blunt. Haksar (2009) the translator of the ancient Sanskrit texts into English, notes: "There are few circumlocutions or polite allusions in its references to sexual and other transgressions, and the language is often blunt, sometimes to the point of crude humour. This may have shocked the pioneering historians of Sanskrit literature. Indologist Winternitz (1927), who acknowledged the *Shuka Saptapati* as one of 'the most famous and popular narratives of India' warned that its contents 'often verge to pornographical stories and some of them are outright obscene'" (pp. xiii–xiv).

The tales are about the perfidy and unfaithfulness of men and women in their intimate relations. It is striking to see the Sanskrit tales of 12 CE printed in popular publications, often sitting side by side with other erotic booklets on the pavements of cities and towns in India. The stories in Hindi are about relations between men and women printed on cheap paper and with titles "*Kissa Tota-Maina*" or 'Tales of the Parrot and the Starling' or simply "Tota-Maina."

The tales, initially passed down in oral tradition from the 7th Century onward, seem to have been compiled into early written editions in the 12th–13th Century; an illustrated edition was commissioned by Emperor Akbar in the mid-16th century. It came to be put together in Persian as *Dastan-e-Hamir Hamza* in the 10th–11th Century. Pritchett (1991) translated it into English titled "Romance in Urdu Literature: Adventures

DOI: 10.4324/9781003626794-3

from the Dastan of Amir Hamzah." Chapter 5 titled Quissa Tota-Mynah – Tale of the Parrot and the Starling begins with: "It is illustrated with crude line drawings, and its cover displays a picture of the kind that has become traditional for this qissa: the parrot and the mynah talking in the branches of a tree, while two human lovers recline under the tree, listening" (p. 1).

The cover of the book "Dastan-e-Tota Maina" (2016) (Tales of the Parrot and the Starling) follows the aesthetics of popular visual culture. It appears like a literal depiction of the introductory remarks of Pritchett, perhaps offering pointers to certain universality in the shaping of gender relations.

The introductory note by the publisher is titled "Do shabd" (Two Words), a common phrase for introductory speeches at literary gatherings. It describes them as ancient tales which, through the medium of the Parrot and the Starling, present the meeting, the anguish of separation, the loyalty and the unfaithfulness of lovers in an evocative way, touching the hearts of readers. Readers might identify with something in each tale that might evoke a spark that seems to tell their own personal story.

Dastan-e Amir Hamza

An excerpt from a translation from the Persian "Dastan-e Amir Hamza" by Pritchett (1991) into English titled "Romance in Urdu Literature: Adventures from the Dastan of Amir Hamzah" gives a flavour of the tales:

Qissā totā mainā (The Parrot and the Mynah)

By chance, one day a parrot, a victim of storms and rain, very anxious, came and sat on a tree to pass his time of trouble. On that same tree was the dwelling place of a mynah (starling).

When the mynah saw the parrot seated on her own tree, she said with great anger, "Oh Parrot! Why have you sat on my tree? Get away from here, and go to some other tree."

Hearing these words, the parrot said, "Oh Mynah! What harm am I doing you? Having passed the night on a branch, at dawn I'll go to my own place."

Upon hearing these words, the Mynah said, "If you say it a thousand times, I still won't agree, because I have great hatred for the race of men. In the whole universe there is no race as pitiless as that of men."

Hearing the mynah's bitter words, the parrot became angry, and said, "What surprising thing is this, that you call men heartless! Indeed, everybody says that the race of women is very heartless and uncompassionate, because some poet has said, No one knows women's wiles, ... Therefore, Mynah! The heartless race is that of women. *There is no other race as true to its word and honest in speech as that of men.* What such defect have you seen in men, that you hate them?"

Then the mynah said, "Oh Parrot! The things for which I hate men, I'll tell you in a dastan. You pay attention and listen" (p. 1).

A story told by the mynah about the perfidy of men is followed by a tale told by the Parrot about the deceitful nature of women.

The tales have the flavour of an adversarial setting – much like a court setting, with each side trying to marshal material to prove the culpability of the other side. The tales seem to be designed to sow seeds of mistrust, deceit and friction between the sexes.

Seventy tales of the parrot

The loaded setting of the Seventy Tales of the Parrot itself gives us an idea of the implicit attitude towards women. A woman's husband is away and she is fixing up a rendezvous with another man. She wrings the neck and almost kills the mynah who admonishes and advises her not to go. On query by the parrot as to where she is going, Haksar notes: (2009) "O king of parrots, I am on my way to find out what it is like to have another man as my lover" (p. 5). The parrot seemingly encourages her, having witnessed the fate of the mynah: "Go to your lover, my beauty," the bird replied. "Afterwards you can listen to this long story if your pretty eyes are still interested." The parrot's words filled her with curiosity, and she stayed back at home. The bird then told her a story." (p. 6). This pattern is repeated 69 times till the return of the husband. The story is representative of the genre. The woman is adamantly trying to get a lover and is somehow lured into not fulfilling the desire. The woman is not shown as remorseful or having turned over a new leaf. The stories seem not to push the triumph of the "faithful" – "good side" of men and women. The next story tells us about the irremediable murderous and greedy side of men with a similar lack of reform or remorse.

First Tale as told by the Mynah

The format of tale within a tale is followed. A story by the mynah about the perfidy of men is followed by a story by the parrot about the unfaithfulness of women.

Ahmad Ali marrying the daughter of a sweeper

Ahmad Ali, the handsome son of a rich merchant, after being on the road a couple of kilometers felt thirsty. On reaching a village, he saw a sweeper's beautiful daughter, swooned and fell unconscious. A crowd collected, sprinkled water and Ali revived and insisted on marrying her. People including the girl's father advised him about difference in caste and status, but to no avail. The father got his daughter married to Ahmad Ali. After some days, he remembered his parents and wanted to go back. The father of the daughter sent them off with riches and ornaments. On the way, Ali thought, "My parents will feel bad at this alliance." He cut her up with knives and threw her into the well. He reached his parents' house with the riches, claiming he had earned them and lived luxuriously.

In the meantime, the injured wife was rescued by a traveller who had gone to the well to draw water. The wife did not reveal the acts of her husband and said robbers had knifed her, thrown her in a well and taken away her riches. She said that the fate of the husband was not known to her. The woman reached her parents' house and related the story of robbery while protecting her parents from knowledge of the crimes her husband had committed.

Meanwhile, Ahmad Ali spent off all the money in a couple of months. Then thought he would go and tell his father-in-law that a son had been born to the daughter, and the father-in-law would give him more riches. Ali on reaching the in-laws house saw his wife sitting there. He panicked and thought, "They will kill me now." The wife calls him dishonest and a scoundrel but reveals that she has not disclosed his evil deeds to her parents and still considers him as her husband. Ali was warmly received and wined and dined. After some days, he expressed a wish to go back to his parents, the wife expresses anxiety, gets reassured and the sequence of events is repeated. Ali again stabs her with knives, takes away the ornaments and leaves her to die. In the tale, the wife is again rescued and reaches home.

These are not tales telling us of the society of the past, and we can see the impact in shaping the psyche and present social attitudes and practices. Much like Ahmad Ali, in real life 6,100 wives were killed for dowry in 2023, the last year for which the data by the National Crime Records Bureau (NCRB) is available. There was a 14% increase in dowry-related crimes and 15,000 cases were registered.[1] Much like the wife's father in the tale who sent them off with ornaments and riches, the father of the bride sends off the daughter with the handing over cash, car, ornaments, furniture and household items referred to as "dowry." The dowry murders are the result of beatings and torture of the woman with demands to bring more money and riches from her father.

Matrix of the tales

The underpinning or subtext of the tales seems to be men's greed and perfidy and women's propensity to be unfaithful, prey to temptation and on the whole lacking in personal ethics. There is perhaps a commonality in certain male and female attitudes in every culture impacting relations with their own specific materials and factors shaping the psyche. The universality is brought home in a rather striking way through Freud's (1925) observations, "Character traits which critics of every epoch have brought up against women – that they show less sense of justice than men, that they are less ready to submit to the great exigencies of life, that they are more often influenced in their judgments by feelings of affection or hostility – all these would be amply accounted for by the modification in the formation of the superego which we have inferred above" (p. 258).

The wife's covering up of the fact of Ali having cut her up, by spinning a yarn of robbery resonates with a hundred stories 'of having fallen down the stairs' to explain bruises in cases of beatings by the husband in domestic abuse cases in courts. The notion of preserving family honour by keeping secrets is a running theme in cases of familial abuse. The influence of the tales in shaping the psyche and impacting gender relations in India till the present takes us to the next section.

Love to Rage

Incidents of "love" turning into rage and revenge culminating in throwing of acid or murderous attacks are often in the news in India. An acid attack involves the intentional throwing of any corrosive substances or any such chemical on a person to cause harm. Such attacks result in severe burns and permanent disfigurement, particularly of the face, often leading to visual impairment, hearing loss and long-term physical disability. The attack results in deep psychological trauma, social stigma and isolation. Rejection of a marriage proposal, non-reciprocation of love and suspicion of infidelity seem to be the main triggers for acid attacks on women. According to the NCRB, 207 acid attacks were reported in India in 2023, up from 202 in 2022 and 176 in 2021, along with 65 attempted attacks (Dristhiias, 2026).[2]

A few sample news reports of incidents are heard from Delhi, Mumbai and Bengaluru, the three major cities in the North, West and Southern region of India, and convey the spread and texture of the dynamics at play.

JNU student attacks classmate with axe, dies after suicide attempt

In a shocking incident, a 23-year-old student died by suicide after attacking a woman classmate with an axe at Jawaharlal Nehru University (JNU). (India Today Online. 2013).

The young woman battling for life shared, "he would be furious if he found me with friends or in a meeting. I had to answer him for every move I made, even if I was just going to the library."

Another woman student attacked in JNU

In another incident in the same campus in August 2013, a student Abhinendra slapped, tried to strangle and push a young woman in front of a moving vehicle.[3] Apparently, the victim-survivor and the perpetrator Abhinendra were former classmates and in a relationship which the young woman had ended (The Hindu 2013).

"Preeti Rathi acid attack in Mumbai: Man convicted for murder"[4]

A special women's court on Tuesday convicted 25-year-old Delhi resident Ankur Panwar for the murder of 23-year-old Preeti Rathi in May 2013. Panwar threw acid on Rathi's face, as he was jealous of her success and because she had spurned his advances (Hindustan Times 2016).

"Acid attack: Women at the receiving end"[5]

A major acid attack took place in the Bengaluru City in 1999, when a man threw the acid as an act of revenge after Haseena turned down his marriage proposal (DHNS2012).

In a series of incidents in the city on 12 August 2002 when Rajesh, a school dropout, threw acid on Shruti, 16, while she was returning home at Shakambari Nagar. In a third incident, a Fairoz forced his wife Hina Fatima to consume a drink laced with sulphuric acid on 8 August 2007 and threw the acid on her. On 21 October 2008, Rakesh allegedly splashed sulphuric acid on Karthika Parameswaran, a final year LLB student of Bishop Cotton Women's Law College, after she rejected his marriage proposal.

There seems to be a refusal to see any interconnections between the present incidents of violence against women and the impact of the oral and written tales on the psyche and texture of men-women relations in India. A distancing and avoiding seeing the links between the behaviour of the characters in the tales with the existence of similar attitudes and actions in contemporary society.

The English translation of *Shukta Saptapati* by Haksar (2009) was received by the press with reviews replete with phrases like 'entertaining social documentation of how men and women lived in ancient India' or 'delighted by the earthiness of the 15th Century text'. Current-day media reports of crimes of passion and violence against women bear a similar lascivious voyeurism, inuring readers against such crimes.

Running streams of legends, tales, movies and songs

The present work seeks to explore the running thread from the ancient tales to contemporary popular cinema in the making and shaping of the psyche and the impact on the dynamics of men-women relations today.

Love at first sight

Laila-Majnu

Laila-Majnu is one of the most popular legends in the Indian subcontinent as well as in Central Asia, with more than half-a-dozen cinematic versions in Hindi, Urdu, Bengali and other languages. The place of this legend in the popular imagination has also crossed over into divinity: there is a "*Laila-Majnu ki mazar*" – the mausoleum of *Laila-Majnu* in Binjaur village in the state of Rajasthan in India. An annual fair is held on 14th June and in a continuing tradition, newlyweds and couples come to offer a *chadar* – cloth shawl and seek blessings. "Majnu" derives from Majnoon meaning "mad" and "possessed" epitomizes the exalted notion of love put on a pedestal. The appeal, hold and place in the popular imagination of this variety of love is reflected in the fact the term "Majnu," is part of the spoken lexicon and can be heard in everyday conversations to depict a "love crazed" man, driven crazy by unfulfilled love.

The stanzas of the epic by Nizami written in 1188, even in translation, manage to convey the texture of the emotions evoked by the legend:

> *"One single glance the nerves to frenzy wrought,*
> *One single glance bewilder'd every thought."*
> (p. 16)

> *"But Oh! when separation came*
> *More brightly glow'd his ardent flame."*
> (p. 17)

> *"And maddened with excessive grief,*
> *In the lone desert he sought relief."*
> (p. 18)

The continuing appeal of the legend is reflected in a contemporary retelling of the tale in the film *Aaja Nachle* (Come Dance) in 2007 and *Laila-Majnu* released in 2018. Nayak (2025) writing of the 2018 film and yearnings for fusion observes "His [Majnu] obsession transcends the mere physical presence of Laila (Triptii Dimri), evolving into an all-consuming yearning for an idealized, almost abstract, beloved. This mirrors the Sufi belief that earthly love can serve as a crucial stepping stone toward comprehending and experiencing divine love, a realm where the individual self ultimately merges with the universal."

The Oedipal themes of envy, jealousy and possessiveness are very much at play in the *Laila-Majnu* story. However, it is perhaps the earlier pre-Oedipal longings of fusion and the intolerableness of separation that form the core of the appeal.

In fact, Plato offers an explanation for feeling of emptiness with eternal yearnings for fusion and in the play Symposium 360 BCE, Aristophanes seeking to explain the search for completeness in love declaims, "In the second place, the primeval man was round, his back and sides forming a circle; and he had four hands and four feet, one head with two faces, looking opposite ways, set on a round neck and precisely alike; also four ears, two privy members, and the remainder to correspond." Zeus, the King of Gods in Greek mythology to weaken splits them and each 'half' forever, seeks the other to feel whole. The yearnings are reflected in popular phrases like "we are two bodies and one soul." The vision of Majnu, the "possessed one" roaming across the scorching desert, wild and disheveled with clothes torn to threads in a delirium, seems to be the very picture of pre-Oedipal strivings of fusion. Perhaps, the strong pull of the saga and the unique place in popular imagination lie in the unconscious resonance of our own yearnings for banishing feelings of hollowness, emptiness and incompleteness in eternal pursuit of feeling whole and complete.

Shakuntala-Dushyant

It is fairly common in campuses for young men who have never spoken a word to the 'object' of their desire, but have "fallen in love" and declared a young woman as "theirs" and get into fights with others for having talked to "their" girl. The legend of Shakuntala-Dushyant is emblematic of the template of love-at-first sight reflected in legends and gathas that impact gender relations today. India is also referred to as "Bharat" and in fact, Article 1(1) of the Constitution of India states: "India, that is Bharat, shall be a union of states." It is believed 'Bharatvarsa' or a unified India/ Bharat is named after Bharata, the son of King Dushyant. King Dushyant on a hunting trip meets Shakuntala, falls in love at first sight and they get married. The King returns to his place with the promise to call her there and forgets. Shakuntala is pregnant and suffers but the tale has a happy ending. The rest of the details need not detain us here for the purposes of this work. It has been immortalized as "Abijnan-Shakuntalam" by Kalidasa 4th-5th Century CE, considered as one of the greatest poets in India. It is a seven-act play and was probably written between the third and sixth centuries.

In the tale, the forgetting by Dushyant is attributed to a curse by the Sage Durvasa.

In fact, the story is illustrative of the nature of love at first sight – shallow, delusionary and ephemeral. It is not a process of spending time with each other getting to know the person as an individual with various facets to them. It is like a trick of mirrors and we see the other person as a reflection of our own projections and not as a real person. Kings and Queens got married with much pomp and show. Dushyant was a King and takes Shakuntala as a commoner, meets her in the forest, performs some gesture with no witnesses, impregnates her, departs and forgets her. In the tale as it unfolds, it is revealed that Shakuntala is the daughter of a celestial nymph who has gone back to heaven. Shakuntala was brought up in an ashram, led a simple life, unlike royalty and is often referred to as "hermit-girl." In Kalidasa's tale, Shakuntala arrives in court, Dushyant treats her as a common, desperate woman claiming to be his wife and she leaves in despair.

SAK: (Aloud) O descendant of Puru, it is indeed, becoming of you, having at first having in that manner deceived this person, naturally simple minded, after a formal agreement in the hermitage, thus to disown her now!

KING: (Closing his ears) Heaven Forbid! Why do you seek to sully your family, and to degrade this person also, as a river, washing away its banks, does to make its waters turbid, and to uproot the tree on the bank? (pp. 181 and 183).

Shakuntala reminds him of the incident of coaxing together a little fawn to drink water, but it falls on deaf ears, and is accused by the King of being a cunning woman.

In the Mahabharata Vana Parva (Book 3), Section CXVII. Internet Sacred Text Archive version of the story, there is no curse or ring and it is about social recognition and truth, she rebukes the king for his lack of truthfulness.

> This is your son, O King. You must anoint him crown prince, just as you promised before, when we met.

When the king heard her, although he remembered her, he said: "I do not remember. To whom do you belong, you wicked hermit-woman? I do not remember a union with you for virtue, love, and wealth. Either go or stay, or do whatever you wish."

When he said this, the sweet hermit-girl half fainted from shame and grief, and stood stiff as a pillar. ....

She seemed to meditate a moment, overcome by grief and anger. She gazed at her husband, then spoke passionately: "O shameless king, although you know, why do you say, 'I do not know', like any other ordinary man?"

Dushyant said: "I do not know the son born of you, Shakuntala. Women are liars. Who will believe what you say? Are you not ashamed to say these incredible things, especially in my presence? You wicked hermit-woman, go!" (pp. 100–101).

Love at first sight to captivated by reflection in mirror

Padmavati and Alauddin Khilji

The story has been immortalized in the epic poem *Padmavat* by *Sufi* poet Malik Muhammad Jayasi in 1540 CE and is a fictionalized retelling of the siege of Chittor by the Delhi Sultan ***Alauddin*** Khilji in 1303. The poem is allegorical with deeper spiritual meaning and a brief summary will suffice for present purposes.

Khilji lays siege to the fort of Chittor and asks for a glimpse of Queen Padmavati. A compromise is reached that Khilji would see Padmavati's reflection in a mirror. On seeing the reflection, Khilji was captivated by her beauty and decides that he won't leave without taking her to Delhi and a war follows. In the face of imminent defeat and victory of Khilji, Padmavati dies by self-immolation to save her "honour" and that of her handmaids, lest they be violated by the victorious army.

The appeal of the story seems eternal and recounted in households and the popularity can be gauged from the fact that a film titled "*Padmavat*" (2018) was made starring popular stars of Hindi cinema.[6]

Bewitched love and star crossed lovers

The universal appeal of bewitched love and star crossed lovers is reflected in myths, legends and tales across cultures. The story of Romeo and Juliet heads the pack in the English-speaking world. Lancelot and Guinevere, Anthony and Cleopatra, Orion and Artemis, Tristan and Iseult, Paris and Helena, Orpheus and Eurydice are some relatively well-known tales. An additional allure is the presence of some token presence of the ill-fated love visible today, which pulls at our heartstrings. In Pyramus and Thisbe, the lovers fix up to meet near the mulberry tree with white berries and run away. Pyramus seeing a bloodied cloak, thinks Thisbe has been eaten by a lion and kills himself and his blood spurts on the mulberry tree. Thisbe returns to the spot and in turn kills herself. The mulberry tree has red berries as a sign of their love. In the Aztec myth of Popocatépetl and Iztaccíhuatl, the princess dies of grief thinking Popocatépetl is dead. He carries her body to the mountain and lights a torch in her memory. The gods turn them into a pair of volcanoes near Mexico City. The Chinese valentine day story has the weaver girl on one side of the Milky Way and the cowherd on other side.

Stalking and Possessiveness As "Love" On Screen

The Indian film industry is the largest in the world, producing 1,500–2,000 films every year in more than 20 languages. Though the revenue generated is not comparable to that of Hollywood, it is also the largest film industry in terms of the number of tickets sold, with 3.5 billion tickets sold annually (compared to Hollywood's 2.6 billion tickets sold annually, Mitra, Nivesh – Global Scenario).[7] Cinema in India has a significant impact on popular culture and people's psyche.

The impact of the "bad" influence of Hindi Cinema popularly referred to as Bollywood, the 'B' standing for the city of Bombay, the location of a large number of film studios, seem to have been taken judicial recognition by a court of law in far-away Australia as a mitigating factor diminishing culpability of the perpetrator.

Bollywood's "bad" influence helps escape stalking conviction in 2015

Sandish Baliga, an Indian man staying in Australia, was accused of stalking two women, texting, calling excessively and began referring to himself as their boyfriend. The 32-year-old security guard maintained that Bollywood movies contributed to his belief that a woman would eventually fall in love with a man if he pursued her enough. The lawyer submitted to the court that it was "quite normal behaviour" for Indian men to pursue women in a similar way and Baliga did not realize his actions could be classed as criminal.

The Hobart magistrate Michael Hill (2015) agreed that Baliga's cultural background helped explain why he did not appreciate the seriousness of his actions. Mr Hill adjourned the complaint without conviction for five years on condition that Baliga should display good behaviour over that period (Hindustan Times. 2015).[8]

Mr. Baliga took the plea of the "bad" influence of Bollywood movies, but Hindi is not the only or even the main language of Indian cinema. There is no centralized or accurate system of accounting for the number of films made, but it is estimated that Bollywood accounts for approximately 17% of films produced in India. Galalite Screens, an industry blog, notes "On an average, India produces a mind boggling number of 1,900 films a year – of which Bollywood accounts for approximately 340 films. The bulk of the rest come from the Tamil, Telugu, Malayalam, Kannada, Marathi, Bengali, Punjabi and Gujarati languages." The present work is focusing on Hindi cinema as illustrative, while acknowledging that the films made in several other languages in India propagate similar notions of "love." For example, the film "*Stalker – A Love Story*," a film made in Kannada, has been dubbed in Hindi and marketed as "Full Hindi Movie" in the advertisement.

Similarly, the Hindi film *Kabir Singh* (2019) is a remake of the Telugu film *Arjun Reddy* (2017). The male protagonist is shown as cool and slapping the female actor is presented as a form of intense "love." The director removes all doubts about the perspective on intimate partner violence presented on the screen by declaring that the liberty to slap each other is a sign of love in couple relationships. The hero chooses the friends his girlfriend can have, denying her any agency. The film also has a scene where the hero threatens a woman to undress at knifepoint. The film has a "happy" ending where the couple reunites, sending the central message of the film of abusive relations as "passionate love."

Journey from teasing to slapping

Chalti-ka-naam gaadi, 1958

(trans.) "That which rolls is called a car"

The film *Chaliti-ka-naam gaadi,* 1958 has the iconic Kishore Kumar and Madhubala as the lead male and female protagonists. The trope of irritating, playfully teasing and annoying a woman to win her over is at full play here. The male actor hates women due to the past heartbreak of his elder brother and mocks the female lead. The woman comes to get the car fixed and the hero sings the song "*Ek ladki-bheegi-bhagi si*" – "A girl soaking wet" while repairing it. The song was and remains wildly popular till today and perhaps, the subliminal message of a wet and frustrated woman contributes to its appeal. The plot includes a scene where the male lead forces the heroine to confess her love for him. The film ends with the "boy" getting the "girl." It is just the kind of film that the Australian Magistrate (2015) accepted as a mitigating factor as having influenced Mr. Baliga in the belief that annoying and harassing a woman brings success in "love" and therefore did not send him to prison for five years.

Kashmir-ki-Kali, 1964

(trans.) "Blossom of Kashmir"

The classic films of Hindi cinema are textbook illustrations of the "not taking a woman's 'No'" for an answer. In the film *Kashmir-ki-Kali* (1964) the hero is shown riding roughshod over her expressions of annoyance. The male lead Shammi Kapoor known for his roles with a trademark "teasing" personality, relentlessly pursues the female lead donning disguises to come near her; performing wild exaggerated antics to get her attention; and obstructing her way to force a conversation and pushing for a commitment to marriage. The film is interspersed with songs with over-the-top exaggerated flattery and wild antics:

"Ye *chand sa roshan chehra, zulfon ka rang sunhara;*
Ye jheel si neeli ankhen, koi raj chipa hai gehra;
Tariff karun kya uski, jisne tujhe banaya"

Trans. English:

"Face lighted up like the moon, with golden colored braids;
Eyes blue as a lake, hiding some deep mystery;
What praise shall I lavish, on the one who has created you."

The lyrics entertain as well as pull at our heartstrings pining for such love and we are seamlessly seduced into the trope of teasing as playful romance in the film.

Sholay, 1975

(trans.) Flames

The heroine Hema Malini, referred to popularly as "Dream Girl" in India, plays the character *Basanti* and drives a "*tonga*"-horse carriage. The muscular hero Dharmendra playing the character *Veeru* jumps on and grabs her from behind. She fights him off and knocks him off the tonga. He climbs aboard again and accompanied by wild antics belts out the song whose lyrics go:

> *"Koi hasina jab rooth jati hai to, aur bhi hasin ho jati hai."*

> (trans.)
> When a beautiful girl is upset, she becomes even more beautiful.

In a later scene, the hero climbs on to a high water tank and threatens to jump off and kill himself as a pressure tactic to get her to marry him.

Even after the passage of half-a-century, the *Basanti-Veeru* scene in the horse carriage has a cult status as a romance sequence in India. The fact that in real life Dharmendra and Hema Malini got married, even though Dharmendra was already married, has only added to the appeal of the scene.

Deewana mujh sa nahi, 1990 has the male lead Ajay in love with his colleague Anita who thinks of him as a friend and is engaged to another man and the wedding is to take place soon. Ajay believes Anita loves him and begins preparations for his wedding with her and gets wedding invitation cards printed. Anita tries to take steps to check Ajay's obsessive love and in the process realizes Ajay's true love and her love for him, and the happy ending of the film has both of them ending up with each other.

Vetticad (2018), speaking of a scene of seduction of the warrior Avantika in the movie *Bahubali* (2015), one of the highest earners initially released in Telugu and Tamil in 2015 and later dubbed into Hindi and Malayalam, writes, "Enraged at the assault, she takes off in search of the offender. When they finally meet face to face, he grabs her, and then comes a sexual dance as he pushes and pulls her about, unties her hair against her will, strips her of her practical fighter's clothing and skilfully transforms the rest of her outfit into more 'feminine' garb. He forcibly smears natural dye on her lips to redden them and lines her eyes with the essence of crushed berries. At this point, she glimpses her transformed self in a sheet of water, and quivers coyly before their dance continues. She finally falls asleep in his arms." The taming of a woman warrior into a feminine stereotype of attire, appearance and behaviour is depicted as "love," with no discussion about consent.

The movies *Deewangi*, 2002, *Teere Naam*, 2003 and *Sawaariya*, 2007 follow the trope of one-sided instant consuming love of the male protagonist, at times leading to abduction and murder. The movie *Ranjhaana*, 2013 has the male protagonist stalking the female character, ignoring her clear rejection and expression of non-reciprocation and threatening to harm himself. The seedlings of "teasing" and "annoying" as love in 1958 in the movie *Chalti-ka-naam gaadi* have grown over the years into stalking as "love" in the 2013 movie *Ranjhaana* and slapping as "passionate love" in the 2019 movie *Kabir Singh*.

Lilting tunes of possessive love

The lyrics of Bollywood songs sung in mellifluous voices have consciously and unconsciously shaped the idea of romantic love as "possessive love" for generations of Indians. There are lilting tones from an earlier era, like Mukesh's rendition from the 1963 film *Dil hi to hai* (trans. 'It is only the heart'):

"tum agar mujkho na chaho to koi baat nahi,
tum kisa aur ko chahogi to mushkil hogi"

(trans. 'It's ok if you don't want me,
It will be difficult if you want anyone else')

We also have Lata Mangeshkar-Mohammed Rafi's rendition from the 1972 film *Aan-Baan* (trans. Friction):

"tum meri ho mere siva kisi ki nahi"

(trans. 'You are mine and belong to no one but me')

It's a running continuum with Rahat Fateh Ali Khan from the 2012 film *Blood Money* soulfully singing:

"Tere ishq pe, tere waqt pe bas haq hai ik mera,
Teri rooh pe, tere jism pe bas haq hai ik mera"

(trans. 'On your love, on your time I have the sole right,
On your soul, on your time I have the sole right')

Cutting to the present, we have Sachet Tandon from the 2025 film *Sunny Sanskari ki Tulsi Kumari* (trans. "Traditional Sunny's Tulsi Maiden') singing:

"ye such to hai tu hai meri
Kaise chupai ishk ab kya chupana
Aata hai Heere tujhe apna banana?"

(trans. '*It's the truth that you are mine*
How to hide my love, why hide now
O Heere I know how to make you mine')

Possessive Love to Rage and Fury

It seems like a seamless transition and "natural" progression from 'love at first sight' leading to 'teasing and annoying as love', progressing to 'slapping as passionate love' and culminating in extreme possessiveness and murderous rage.

The interconnections of cinema impacting popular psyche and the filmmakers' claim that the movies portray social realities is like the 'chicken and the egg' conundrum which can run endlessly in a loop. The plots of a few illustrative films, perhaps, may manage to convey the flavor of the Bollywood offerings on the subject.

Darr (trans. Fear)

In the film *Darr*, 1993, the college student Kiran is stalked by an obsessive man who takes her photos secretly and breaks into her home. The stalker projects Kiran's 8-foot pictures on each wall of his house and practises the pickup line – *"Tu haan kar, ya na kar, tu hai meri Kiran"* (trans. "You say Yes, or you say No, you are mine Kiran"). Kiran marries her fiancée and the stalker carves her name on his chest with a knife to "claim" her. The stalker befriends Kiran's family plotting to kill the husband and abduct her. The climax has the stalker stabbing the husband who manages to shoot and kill the stalker. The stalker is played by Shah Rukh Khan, superstar and quintessential romantic hero of Hindi cinema and the song "जादू तेरी नज़र/खुश्बू तेरा बदन/.... तू हाँ कर या ना कर/तू है मेरी किरण ..." (trans. "Your eyes are magic/your body is fragrance/....you say yes or say no/you are mine Kiran") is a widely popular song described as a timeless hit. The stalker may have been killed in the end, but his obsession contributes to the glamorization of stalking as 'love'.

Anjaam (trans. Consequence)

In the movie *Anjaam*, 1994, a wealthy businessman Vijay gets infatuated with an air hostess, Shivani, who repeatedly rejects him. Shivani marries and has a daughter. The businessman murders her husband and covers it up by bribing the police. Shivani again rejects Vijay who beats her up and frames her for attempted murder leading to her imprisonment. Vijay accidentally runs his car over and kills the daughter. The film ends with both Vijay who has been stabbed by Shivani, hanging from a cliff and both falling to their death.

The film has the top glamorous stars of Hindi cinema and Shah Rukh Khan playing the stalker won the "Filmfare Best Villain Award" for the performance. Shivani is played by Madhuri Dixit who got the "Filmfare Best Actress Award" the same year for another film. Shah Rukh Khan and Madhuri Dixit made an "amazing" pair and the dying together in the movie *Anjaam* and both receiving awards in the same event pulls at romantic heartstrings.

Daraar (trans. Fissure)

In the movie *Daraar*, 1996, the husband Vikram has an intensively possessive love for his wife Priya. The husband gets enraged at any show of independence by the wife and beats her up. Priya fakes her death in a boating accident to escape the physical abuse. She meets Raj who falls in love with her and they decide to marry. Vikram learns that she is with another man. An enraged Raj then tracks them down, gets Raj falsely imprisoned and tries to kill Priya. Raj escapes and drowns the husband in a bathtub. Vikram survives, pushes Raj and chases Priya. In the final scene, Vikram's foot is stuck in railway track and Priya, despite the abuse and attempt to kill her, tries to save him. At the last minute, Vikram pushes her away before the train hits him declaring "Today, I free you from all bonds." Thus even as the film ends with the husband's death, the message is loud and clear as to the continuing ownership of the husband who tried to kill and who an act of magnanimity chooses to "free" the wife of all bonds.

Narcissistic Injury and Rage

> The ego, furthermore, increasingly surrenders its reasoning capacity to the task of rationalizing the persisting insistence on the limitlessness of the power of the grandiose self: it does not acknowledge the inherent limitations of the power of the self, but attributes its failures and weaknesses to the malevolence and corruption of the uncooperative archaic object.
>
> Kohut (1972) (p. 396)

> Talk not to me of blasphemy, man; I'd strike the sun if it insulted me.
>
> Captain Ahab in Moby Dick Melville (1851) (p. 131)

Kohut's postulation of abandoning reason, feeling powerful and blaming the other for one's failures can be seen at play in the protagonists of the three films *Darr, Anjaam* and *Darrar* plotting to kill the object of their love.

Hindu mythology abounds in stories of perceived slights, evoking rage, curses and at times killings by Sages and other holy figures. They are revered as extraordinary beings who through self-discipline, penance and devotions acquire magical powers and their boons and curses come true for ordinary mortals.

Quicksilver anger Durvasa

Children in Hindu households grow up listening to stories of the quick to anger Sage *Durvasa* with his mercurial temper, which was unleashed at every perceived slight. The sage habitually cursed human beings and did not spare even the gods. We would listen with anxiety imagining the sage turning up at our households and cursing us to horrible fates. A few illustrations conjure up the flavour of the Durvasa phenomenon.

Curse on Rukmini

The God Krishna, the King of Dwaraka and his Queen Rukmini invited Durvasa for a meal. Durvasa consented on the condition that Krishna and his wife Rukmini pull his chariot instead of horses. Rukmini felt exhausted and thirsty, Krishna struck his toe in the soil and Ganga water sprang forth. Rukmini drank the water without his permission. The Sage cursed her with separation from her husband for 12 years. As children we quailed at the thought that even mundane everyday acts like drinking water could result in being cursed to undergo agonies.

In Skanda Purana *VII (*Ancient Indian Tradition and Mythology, Volume 55) the verses go as follows:

Verse 48: Durvasa said: "O Rukmini of beautiful face, since you have drunk water without seeking my permission, you will undoubtedly become addicted to the habit of drinking [water/liquids] constantly."

Verse 49: "Since you drank the water without taking the yoke off your shoulders and without asking me, O fair-faced one, you shall suffer separation from Krishna."

Verse 50: Having spoken thus, the Brahmana (Durvasa), his eyes red with anger, got down from the chariot and sat upon the ground.

Verse 51: Being thus cursed, the Goddess (Rukmini) began to weep loudly, saying, "O Krishna, how shall I stay without you, being distressed by separation?"

Dushyant-Shakuntala

In the Dushyant-Shakuntala story (Kalidasa. 4th – 5th Century CE 1969) mentioned above, it is as a result of the curse of Durvasa that Dushyant forgets her. Shakuntala day dreaming of Dushyant fails to notice the arrival of Durvasa, who at this perceived insult, curses her that the person she was thinking of would forget her entirely and in the way of mythical stories, it comes about to be true

Reducing wife Kandali to ashes

Durvasa in an argument with his wife Kandali got angry and cursed her with getting burnt to ashes. Kandali instantly turned into a pile of ashes.

Brahmavaivarta Purana, Prakriti-Khanda. (2003)

- **Verse 53:** Durvasa tolerated more than one hundred insults from his wife, keeping his promise to her father, Sage Aurva.
- **Verse 55:** Unable to control his rising anger after she exceeded this limit, he cursed her: *"Become a pile of ashes!."*
- **Verse 56:** At his word, she was instantly consumed by fire and reduced to ashes.

Innumerable myths tell us about various aspects of human nature and are in the nature of action-stories. The grandiosity of the self, the fragility of the ego, the propensity to perceive behaviour of the other as insult resulting in narcissistic injury and the inability to contain emotions especially in the nature of anger and fury are brought home time and again. The protagonists in the stories are evolved superior beings like sages and at times gods and perhaps give us a clue as to the difficulties in engaging with these parts for ordinary mortals.

The relevance of the myths in the shaping of the psyche and impact on behaviour can be seen in a number of incidents in contemporary India. Radhika Yadav, a 25-year-old young state-level woman tennis player coaching aspiring tennis players was shot dead by her father on 10 March 2025 in Gurgaon in Haryana, a state in India. The father despite being financially secure with an independent income felt humiliated by taunts of villagers of living off his daughter's income coaching. Enraged, and unable to contain his fury, her father shot Radhika four times in the back and waist.[9]

The protagonists of bubbling anger bursting into violent fury are mostly male and, perhaps a reflection of society in India. At a mythological level, there is the Goddess Kali who decapitates, wears a garland of severed heads with one foot on the body of her consort Shiva. In everyday life, there is no space for expression of female resentments and anger which builds up and explodes as possession by an evil spirit or ghost. It is only through the device of being possessed by an evil spirit that a woman can hurl abuses, resentments and curses at her husband, mother-in-law, sisters-in-law and sundry other characters. Like Balaji temple in Rajasthan, there are places scattered all over India and people from clusters of villages periodically visit to exorcise the demon and women get a chance to vent out their anger and fury. They can say just about anything as it is evil spirit within them speaking and so they are not to be held accountable for the utterances. After these outbursts, it's back to everyday life with no outlet for resentments and angers. Kakar 1982 takes a closer look at the psychic process at play in Shamans, mystics and doctors.

Rage on steroids

Sage Parshuram and the killing of 21 generations

According to legend, *Parshuram* was the son of Sage Jamadagni and belonged to the priestly *Brahmin* caste. *Parshuram* is literally Ram with an axe. The sage was killed by the sons of the *Kshatriya* warrior caste King Sahastrabahu. *Parshuram* heard the call of his mother, reached the ashram and saw the severed head of his father and 21 cuts on his body. An enraged *Parshuram* took an oath, and wiped off 21 generations of the warrior caste Kshatriyas wielding his axe and filled five lakes with their blood.

Mahabharata – Internet Sacred Text Archive

> *And, O chieftain of the military caste, Rama, the leader of all capable of beating their foes, thrice smote down all the Kshatriya followers of Kartavirya's sons. And seven times did that powerful lord exterminate the military tribes of the earth. In the tract of land, called Samantapanchaka five lakes of blood were made by him.*

In the myth, Jamadagni at a perceived momentary distraction of his wife thinking of another man orders the sons to kill her. *Parshuram*'s elder brothers refuse and are cursed by the father. *Parshuram* beheads his mother and brothers conveying the enmeshing intensity of the father-son relation. The murder of his father, perhaps, was experienced as a deep narcissistic injury threatening the very sense of self of *Parshuram*. That behind the grandiose exterior self, lurked a fragile ego totally dependent on approval and validation by the father to the extent of killing the mother on his orders. The sudden violent death of the father by killing in such a fused bond may have triggered shame, guilt, self-recrimination, inadequacy, perhaps even rage at oneself at not being present and able to protect the father. In such relational dynamics at play, there appears to be no room for healthy mourning. The near-fatal puncturing blow to the sense of self and self-worth needs a murderous fury and revenge on a grand scale by personally beheading 21 generations wielding the axe in an attempt to resurrect and prop up the grandiose self.

Rage to Killing

The myths and stories still related in households are like pointers towards our uncontrollable rages and furies and the difficulties in containing and managing emotions. The eruptions of such murderous rages into violence and murder in an intimate love relationship periodically find their way in the newspapers. The love story of the Shradha and Aftab belonging to different faiths, and defying society to live together is the very picture of true romance.

Shradha Walkar murder case[10]

Shradha and Aftab met at a call centre in 2018 and love blossomed in the inter-religious Hindu-Muslim relationship. Shradha's parents were against the relationship because they belonged to different religions (BBC 2022).

Shradha was a bold, confident woman with the Instagram handle – "That Short Rebel" who told her mother that she wanted to stay in live-in relationship with Aftab and took up a place Mumbai. Lurking behind the picture book façade was the reality of Aftab's rage and violence. The couple shifted to Delhi in 2022, and soon thereafter Aftab strangled Shradha to death. A trained chef, Aftab cut her into 35 pieces and stored the parts in polythene bags in the fridge and over a period of six months disposed them in the forested areas of Delhi and Gurgaon. The gruesome crime came to light only about six months later as a consequence of Shradha's father filing a missing person's complaint (The New Indian Express 2023).

The case is perhaps emblematic of the love and rage in intimate love relationships. A series of similar incidents surfaced in the media. The Nikki Yadav-Sahil Gehlot Case (Delhi, 2023) – a 23-year-old woman Nikki Yadav was allegedly strangled by her partner, Sahil Gehlot, who then stuffed her body into a refrigerator in his roadside eatery[11]; the murder of a 32-year old woman by her live-in partner, who chopped her body and boiled the parts in a cooker dubbed by the press as the Mira Road "Cooker" Murder (2023)[12] and the murder of a 29-year-old woman chopped into 50 pieces by a 30-year-old man in Bengaluru. The parts were found stuffed inside a refrigerator and referred to in the media as the Bengaluru Refrigerator murder (2024) case.[13]

Each of the individuals involved in the incidents come with their own set of circumstances, family history, childhood, adolescence, private inner life and social life. Generalizations as to triggers and motivations may not be possible. The sole consistent factor seems to be the inability to contain anger. The vicissitudes of life throw many challenges including feelings of being slighted, humiliated and insulted evoking anger. As part of the developmental stage of growing up, we learn to contain and to partly process at times the virulent intensity of our emotions to make them more palatable and tolerable to ourselves. In a sense when this process gets thwarted due to various factors, the emotions erupt like a volcano leading to violence. Perhaps, the ego at times is too weak and fragile to contain the impulses raging within the self. A major project of therapy becomes of forming an alliance with the ego to assist in mediating between the Id and the external reality to reach a balance.

The Dynamics of Narcissism and Love

> The subject's narcissism makes its appearance displaced on this new ideal ego, which like the infantile ego, finds itself possessed of every perfection that is of value .... What he projects before him as his ideal is the substitute for the lost narcissism of his childhood in which he was his own ideal.
>
> Freud (1914) (pp. 81–82)

The love reflected in the popular song from the film *Darr* (1993) rendered in a mellifluous tune "You say yes or say no/You are mine" seems to have no space for the "loved object" in a relationship. Even, if at a conscious rationale level we reject the "possessive love" of the song, yet, perhaps it has a subliminal appeal to certain parts of ourselves. Our longings as adults of being "All-Powerful" –perhaps tapping into the feelings of omnipotence experienced as a baby. The infant feels hungry and a breast or bottle appears immediately as if magically created by the baby (Winnicott, 2005). Perhaps, akin to an infant who assumes rights over a soft toy, a blanket, a towel which is "cuddled as well as excitedly loved and mutilated" and "must survive instinctual loving, and also hating and, if it be a feature, pure aggression" (p. 7) – like the protagonist in the song – the dynamic plays out in the "romantic love" relation.

The nurturing breast and the illusion of omnipotence along with the concomitant grandiose self appear to be a necessary developmental stage – the baby experiencing the "good breast." However, at times the baby is hungry and if the breast is not there or is experienced as the frustrating "bad breast," evoking extreme anger, reflected in the coinage of the phrase "infantile rage." It is likely that at times, a baby may feel suffocated and unable to breathe and bites the breast that provides milk, the baby's sustenance. This may get compounded in a culture where the male child at times is suckled at the breast till a fairly late age, as evidenced in the course of my clinical practice, when in fact there is no nurturing milk in the mother's breast. This may be experienced as being "smothered" by the breast and may feed into the little boy's anxieties and fears about being annihilated and incorporated by a powerful "devouring mother."

Klein (1946) notes "Therefore in addition to the divorce between a good and a bad breast in the young infant's phantasy, the frustrating breast-attacked in oral-sadistic phantasies-is felt to be in fragments; the gratifying breast, taken in under the dominance of the sucking libido, is felt to be complete" (pp. 5–6). Ideally, the growing baby successfully integrates the "bad breast" and the "good breast" – the "nurturing mother" and the "frustrating absent mother." In the context of the integration of the "good" mother and the "bad" mother, Roy (2025) in her autobiography speaking of her mother pithily articulates "She was my shelter and my storm" (Back cover). The "Fairy Godmother" and the "Evil Stepmother" of "Cinderella" in the story seem like a textbook illustration of the split between the good and the bad. Perhaps, an epilogue to the fairy tale, a sort of coming of age of Cinderella to the realization that the "Kind" Godmother and the "Cruel" Stepmother is the same person.

Oscillations between Omnipotence and Nothingness

It is likely that the integration of the "Kind Godmother" and the "Cruel Stepmother" does not proceed in a seamless way according to the hypothesized developmental stages. Perhaps, it is a lifelong engagement where we struggle with the splits, projections and projective identifications in our social, political and personal lives. Johar-Krizan (2015), based on four studies comparing narcissistic vulnerability and grandiosity as predictors of anger and rage, concludes, "Evidence presented here offers strong support for narcissistic vulnerability as the source of narcissistic rage, while also revealing narcissistic grandiosity not to be a potent predictor of reactive or displaced aggression" (p. 796).

There are infinite variations of human feelings and thoughts, however, in about two decades of psychoanalytic therapy practice there appears to be a fairly consistent pendulum like swing between the "I am the greatest" feeling and "I am nothing" paradigm.

A vignette from a clinical session may be able to illustrate this:

The session is at 8 am. B reaches at 8.10 am.

B: I started at 7.45 am from home and reached outside your door at 8.07 am. I drove at high speed 95–97 km per hour from inner lanes and reached.
T:Hmmm
B: No. Not just here. I do this in everything. The time I have to reach a place – at that time I start. Let me tell you about today. *Namaz* (trans. Prayer) is at 5.50 am. I put the alarm for 5.40 am. I woke up. Then thought it *namaz* is at 5.50 am, I will be able to reach – let me sleep a bit more. I reached at 6 am.
T: Like when you have to come for the session at 8 am
B: I should plan that I will get out at 7.30 am and reach at 8 am. At 7.30 am I feel, there is time, I will be able to reach. I feel I will be able to reach in five minutes.
T: Hmm
B: And people will say, 'Oh! How did this happen! How did he manage to do this?'
T: Like in fairy stories, you will suddenly appear.
B: Yes. For an 8 to 9 am meeting, I start at 8 am and reach late. Then I stay there for half an hour. People come, kick me and pass by. They make a fool of me. Use me. Kick me. Make fun of me and proceed onwards. This is my pattern.

In the course of the session, the magical grandiose self who can do amazing things swings to the other side, to the fool who is made fun of and kicked around.

Kohut (1972) succinctly articulates the objectives of therapy, "We shall then be able, as can be observed in the systematic therapeutic analysis of narcissistic personality disturbances, to transform our archaic grandiosity and exhibitionism into realistic self-esteem and into pleasure with ourselves, and our yearning to be at one with the omnipotent self-object into the socially useful, adaptive, and joyful capacity to be enthusiastic and to admire the great after whose lives, deeds, and personalities we can permit ourselves to model our own" (p. 365).

The flip side of magical grandiosity seems to be feelings of being small and insignificant, like being an extra in a crowd scene of a film. A lot of work of the therapeutic process seems to be to move towards the middle ground between "I am the greatest" and "I am not anything." Perhaps, efforts at reality checks and attempts at grounding the flights of fancy leading to suppression of the grandiose omnipotent selves and wishes to be great, famous and the main protagonist in the film may be counterproductive and not a constructive avenue to explore in therapy. It is the playing out of the flights of fancy, the unfolding of the conscious and unconscious fantasies, of experiencing the highs of climbing mountain peaks and exploring the mysterious depths of the oceans which may help the process. Simultaneously, rather than a facile reassurance, perhaps it is the staying, articulating and elaborating the feelings in the nature of smallness and insignificance, which may facilitate the movement towards a stable middle rather than swinging between the two extremes of feeling to be the greatest human on earth and to feeling like a mere speck of dust.

Never the twain of perfidy and giddy love shall meet?

The streams of unfaithfulness, deception, violence, betrayal between men and women run parallel to the flowing currents of Valentine's day, the delights of love and romance. Back in 360 BC, Plato postulated a being that incorporated both sexes with four legs, arms and separate genitals. However, this being was separated by the God Zeus, therefore causing a perennial yearning for the other to feel a sense of completeness. This desire for fusion reflected in current notions of exalted heterosexual love is a thread that has run through men-women relations through the ages and continues to the present times. The perfidy stream runs from oral traditions of the seventh century, through folk tales published in booklets in various languages sold on pavements to impressive looking illustrated manuscripts commissioned by monarchs to pioneering intellectuals like Freud and poets like Wesley. The parallel streams continue to run through plays, television screens and films.

Therapy rooms resound with the cries and frustrations of rosy love crashing on the hard rocks of reality. The lilting tunes of "*Tum mere sath hoge, gum bahut door hoga*" (trans. You'll be with me, sorrow will stay far") prove to be a chimera. The conscious-unconscious longings, the incipient phantasizes that all feelings of emptiness, loneliness, of being flawed and defective would vanish on finding the "loved one" prove to be the search for proverbial mirage of water to quench our thirsts. The longing for the perfect relation where I'll never disappoint the other and the other will never disappoint me and where the other will fulfil my every need, said and unsaid, impacts our relationships. At times, a sense of narcissistic injury at the disappointments and hurts provokes murderous fury towards the "love object." Much like the swings between our grandiose and insignificant selves, the strivings in therapy are to see ourselves and the other as a "real" person with human frailties and flaws and work towards a relationship gently grounded on earth rather than dwelling in the fluffy cloud castles in azure blue skies.

Notes

1 Dowry cases rise by 14% in 2023; over 6,100 women killed: NCRB. The Hindu. 3 October 2025.
2 Acid attacks in India. Dristhiias.com 7 January 2026.
3 Another woman student attacked in JNU. The HINDU. Published – 06 August 2013 02:05 am IST – New DelhiIANS
4 Preeti Rathi acid attack in Mumbai: Man convicted for murder. Hindustan Times. 7 September 2016
5 Acid attack: Women at the receiving end DHNS Last Updated: 23 April 2012.
6 *Padmavat*. Film. 2018. Director – Sanjay Leela Bhansali.
7 Nivesh Mitra – Global Scenario.
8 Bollywood 'bad influence' helps Indian man escape conviction for stalking Aus women. Hindustan Times. 29 January 2015.
Bollywood excuse helps Hobart stalker avoid conviction. 29 January 2015. ABC News.
9 Murdered tennis player Radhika Yadav cremated, father says he was taunted for living off her income. The Hindu. 12 July 2025; Radhika Yadav's Murder: Psychology Of Pride, Patriarchy, And Prejudice. NDTV. 13 July 2025.
Please see section on "Honor Killings" in "Of Gods and Demons: the murderous rage of the ordinary".
10 BBC Shraddha Walkar and Aftab Poonawala: India gripped by gruesome 'fridge murder'. 25 November 2022.
11 Delhi Fridge Murder: Accused To Stay In Judicial Custody For 14 More Days. 22 March 2023. https://www.ndtv.com/delhi-news/nikki-yadav-murder-case-sahil-gehlot-to-stay-in-custody-for-14-more-days-3884827
12 32-Year-Old Murdered In Mumbai, Tree Cutter Used To Chop Body: 10 Points. 8 June 2023. https://www.ndtv.com/india-news/32-year-old-murdered-in-mumbai-tree-cutter-used-to-chop-body-10-points-4105664
13 Home-alone woman found dead in Bengaluru. The Hindu. 22 September 2024.

Bibliography

Acid attack: Women at the receiving end DHNS Last Updated: 23 April 2012 https://www.deccanherald.com/india/karnataka/bengaluru/acid-attack-women-receiving-end-2328320 Retrieved 18th December 2025.
Acid attacks in India. Dristhiias.com. 7th January 2026. https://www.drishtiias.com/daily-updates/daily-news-analysis/acid-attacks-in-india-1 Retrieved 27th February 2026.
Aaja Nachle. 2007. Movie. Director Anil Mehta.
Anjaam. 1994. Movie. Director Rawail, Rahul.
Another woman student attacked in JNU. The Hindu. Published - August 06, 2013 02:05 am IST - New DelhiIANS. https://www.thehindu.com/news/cities/Delhi/another-woman-student-attacked-in-jnu/article4993086.ece#google_vignette Retrieved 9th January 2026.
Arjun Reddy. Movie. 2017. Director Vanga, Sandeep Reddy.
Bahubali. 2015. Movie. Director Rajamouli, SS.
Battle of the Sexes. 2017. Movie. Valerie Faris, Valerie and Jonathan Dayton, Jonathan.

Bollywood 'bad influence' helps Indian man escape conviction for stalking Aus women. influence-helps-indian-man-escape-conviction-for-stalking-aus-women/story-iuoSfczLoZKSbPJKkz6NeK.html Retrieved 19 December 2025.
Brahmavaivarta Purana, Prakriti-Khanda. Chapter 23, Verses 52–56. Translated Shantilal Nagar. 2003. Parimal Publications. Delhi.
Chalti-ka-naam gaadi. 1958. Movie. Director Bose, Satyen.
Cooker Murder (2023). 32-Year-Old Murdered In Mumbai, Tree Cutter Used To Chop Body: 10 Points. 8 June 2023. https://www.ndtv.com/india-news/32-year-old-murdered-in-mumbai-tree-cutter-used-to-chop-body-10-points-4105664
Daraar. 1996. Movie. Director Burmawalla, Abbas and Burmawalla, Mustan.
Darr. 1993. Movie. Director Chopra, Yash.
Dastaan-e-Tota-Maina. 2016. Presentation Govind Singh. New Sadhana Pocket Books. Delhi.
Deewangi. 2002. Movie. Director Bazmee Aneez.
Freud, S. 1914. On Narcissism: An Introduction. Vol. XIX. Revised Standard Edition.
Freud, S. 1925. Some psychical consequences of the anatomical differences between the sexes. Vol. XIX. Revised Standard Edition.
Haksar, A.N.D. 2009. Shuka Saptapati – seventy tales of the parrot. Translated from the Sanskrit by AND Haksar. Rupa Publications India Private Ltd. New Delhi.
Johar, Omesh and Krizan, Zlatan. 2015. Narcissistic Rage Revisited. Journal of Personality and Social Psychology © 2014 American Psychological Association 2015, Vol. 108, No. 5, pp. 784–801. Retrieved 2nd January 2026.
JNU student attacks classmate with axe, dies after suicide attempt. India Today Online. Updated July 31, 2013. https://www.indiatoday.in/india/north/story/delhi-jawaharlal-nehru-university-student-attacks-classmate-with-axe-suicide-172248-2013-07-30 Retrieved 18th December 2025.
Kabir Singh. 2019. Movie. Director Vanga, Sandeep Reddy.
Kakar, S. 1982. Shamans, Mystics and Doctors: A Psychoanalytic Inquiry Into India and Its Healing Traditions. Oxford University Press. Oxford.
Kalidasa. 4th–5th Century CE. Ed. Kale M.R. Tenth Edition 1969. Reprint 1980. Motilal Banarsidass. Indological Publishers and Booksellers. Delhi.
Kashmir-ki-kali. 1964. Film. Director Shakti Samant.
Klein, M. 1946. Notes on some schizoid mechanisms. Klein-M.-1946.-Notes-on-some-schizoid-mechanisms.pdf. Retrieved 6th January 2026.
Kohut, H. 1972. Thoughts on Narcissism and Narcissistic Rage. The Psychoanalytic Study of the Child. Volume 27. Hogarth Press. London.
Mahabharata, Vana Parva (Book 3), Section CXVII. Internet Sacred Text Archive. https://sacred-texts.com/hin/m03/m03117.htm Retrieved 6th January 2026.
Melville, Herman. 1851. Moby Dick. herman-melville-moby-dick.pdf Retrieved 6th January 2026.
Mitra, Nivesh. Global Scenario. https://niveshmitra.up.nic.in/Film.aspx Retrieved 17th February 2026
Nayak, A. 2025. Echoes of Eternity: Philosophical Perspectives on Love in 'Laila Majnu'. The Movie Buff. https://www.themoviebuff.net/2025/06/echoes-of-eternity-philosophical-perspectives-on-love-in-laila-majnu/ Retrieved 30th December 2025.
Ranjhaana. 2013. Movie. Director Rai, Aanand L.
Roy, Arundhati. 2025. Mother Mary Comes To Me. Penguin Random House India. Gurugram.
Sawaariya. 2007. Movie. Director Bhansali, Sanjay Leela.
Sholay. 1975. Movie. Director Sippy, Ramesh.
Shradha Walkar and Aftab Poonawala: India gripped by gruesome 'fridge murder'. BBC. 25 November 2022. https://www.bbc.com/news/world-asia-india-63739683 Retrieved 9th January 2026.

The Shradha Walkar murder. The New Indian Express. 30 April 2023. https://www.newindianexpress.com/cities/delhi/2022/Nov/21/explainer-the-shraddha-walkar-murder-2520521.html Retrieved 9th January 2026.

The Skanda Purana, Part VII (Ancient Indian Tradition and Mythology, Volume 55). Translated by G.V. Tagare. 1995. Motilal Banarsidass Publishing House. Delhi.

Padmavat. 2018. Movie. Director – Bhansali, Sanjay Leela.

Plato. Symposium 360 BCE. Translation Jowett, Benjdamin. 1871. Oxford University Press. https://classics.mit.edu/Plato/symposium.htmlm Retrieved 18th February 2026

Preeti Rathi acid attack in Mumbai: Man convicted for murder. Hindustan Times mumbai-man-convicted-for-murder/story-VOL5yZNIen45cRaavMkcOJ.html Retrieved 18th December 2025.

Pritchett, Franics W. 1991. Quissa Tota – Maina. Chapter 5 - The Romance Tradition in Urdu: Adventures from the Dastan of Amir Hamzah. Columbia University Press.

Teere Naam. 2003. Movie. Director Kaushik, Satish.

Vetticad, Anna am. 2018. The rape of Avantika. Business Line. https://www.thehindubusinessline.com/blink/watch/the-rape-of-avanthika/article64570050.ece Retrieved 31st December 2025.

Winnicott. D.W. 2005. Playing and Reality. Routledge Winnicott Classics. Routledge. Abingdon, Oxon.

Winternitz, M. History of Indian Literature. Calcutta 1927. Trans. Subhadra Jha. 1985. Motilal Banarsidass Publishing House. Delhi.

3 Law and Psychoanalysis

The Logical Meets the Irrational

Making submission before the Supreme Court of India in a petition against the construction of concrete roads in a designated National Wildlife Sanctuary situated in the densely forested Bastar region of India, I was taken aback to find one of the judges trembling with rage. The administration had been digging up gravel and rocks in the sanctuary on the specious plea that the material was not being taken out of the sanctuary and therefore could not be categorized as a non-forest activity. The activities were prohibited under the Wildlife Protection Act, 1972. The submissions were purely legal having little in them to evoke such sound and fury. At the last hearing, the Supreme Court bench had been ready to penalize the government for making a mockery of the conservation laws. The forested area was also the base of a strong Marxist-Leninist-Maoist social movement referred to as "left-wing extremism" and the State Counsel had harped on detonators, mines, mud roads and explosions. Perhaps, the submissions tapped into the judge's anxieties about being torn apart or beheaded by angry mobs; fears of the breakdown of law and order, bloody revolution and being swamped in the quicksand of anarchy. The magnitude of the fury had made his face red and the judge was addressing the legal counsel – in this case me – as if I was an accused before him and had personally planted detonators and mines in the area.

The law was clear, and the submissions made were bland and purely legal in nature, yet intense emotions were evoked in the judge, confronting us with the incontrovertible fact that justice is dispensed by human beings prey to a hundred anxieties, fears, and flights of fancy, arbitrariness and whimsy. This brings us to the heart of the rational and the logical of law colliding with the workings of the human psyche in the strivings for justice. The wildlife conservationist petitioners and I as their lawyer were feeling aggrieved and the phrase of Justice Brennan, one of the most influential United States Supreme Court judges in the area of civil rights "Nothing rankles more in the human heart than a brooding sense of injustice",[1] resonated with us.

DOI: 10.4324/9781003626794-4

Rational and the irrational

In contrast to the logical and the rational, the human psyche is a like a seething cauldron of fears and anxieties, insecurities and prejudices, as well as raging contradictory emotions like love and hate, empathy and cruelty. Freud (1933) observes "The logical laws of thought do not apply in the id, and this is true above all of the law of contradiction" (pp. 65–66). Kakar (1981) drawing parallels between Freud's (1933) approach to id with analogies like "a chaos, a cauldron full of seething excitations" (p. 65) writes "Some Hindu texts draw the metaphor of a monkey, restless by nature, who drinks wine and becomes even more restless. As if this were not enough, he is stung by a scorpion, and – to complete the image of uncontrolled restlessness – a demon enters him." "*Chitta*, in its normal state, is compared to this monkey, drunk with wine, smarting under the scorpion bite and possessed by a demon[2]" (p. 22).

Even a fleeting appearance in the courtroom as a litigant or witness makes visible the foibles and fallibilities of the individual adorning the bench. The judge is at the end of the chain and the extra-legal factors at play are true for all the dramatis personae on the legal stage. It begins with the Draughtsman or Draftsman – the individual who actually formulates the various provisions of a statute and puts down the sections, sub-sections and exceptions in black and white, but who never makes an appearance on the stage. Next in the chain is the Implementer of the law or the Executive, followed by the Investigator, the Prosecutor, the Mediator, the Lawyer and the Judge, each of whom comes with their own respective baggage. As we unfold the layers, invisible biases, prejudices and stereotypes emerge and interact with each other. A number of extra-legal factors like appearance, gender, attire, language, accent and a hundred other minutiae are registered by and impact the psyche. Shukla (2019) explores the baggage carried in terms of biases, prejudices and stereotypes and the impact of extra-legal factors in the Chapter titled "Quest for Justice: psychoanalytical explorations with judges". The exploration is Chapter 5 of the present book titled "Inner world of judges – psychoanalytical explorations.[3]

Irrational impacts rational

The impact of the irrational on seemingly rational decisions can be clearly seen in judicial pronouncements. Parole can be granted to a prisoner on certain grounds before the completion of the sentence imposed by a court of law. The factors to be considered while taking a decision on parole are the prisoner's behaviour, assessment of correctional staff and psychologists, feelings of remorse, chances of committing the offence again, following rules, possibilities of rehabilitation and motivation for reparation, the impact on the victim/survivor, the possibility of influencing or threatening witnesses and the nature of the crime. In addition, events like illness or death in the family, weddings and birth of a child are valid grounds to give temporary parole.

Danziger et al. (2011) observe that "Realists argue that the rational application of legal reasons does not sufficiently explain judicial decisions and that psychological, political, and social factors influence rulings as well (4)." The realist view is commonly caricaturized by the trope that justice is "what the judge ate for breakfast" (5). We empirically test this caricature in the context of sequences of parole decisions made by experienced judges (mean experience = 22.5 years, standard deviation (SD) = 2.5) and, in so doing, demonstrate how extraneous factors can sway highly consequential decisions of expert decision makers.

The Danziger-Levav-Avanaim-Pesso team analysed more than 1000 rulings in 2009 made by two parole boards where eight judges ruled on whether to grant parole-related requests from prisoners in four Israeli prisons. They recorded the chronological order of the rulings relative to two food breaks that the judges took each day – one for a morning snack and the other for a lunch. The percentage of rulings in favour of the prisoners fell gradually from about 65% to nearly zero in each of the three decision-making sessions demarcated by the two breaks. It abruptly leapt back to 65% immediately, after the breaks, suggesting that prisoners whose cases were heard at the start of the day or soon after a break had an advantage over other prisoners.

The team concludes that the findings bolster a view that judicial reasoning is hardly iron clad and observes, "Finally, our findings support the view that the law is indeterminate by showing that legally irrelevant situational determinants—in this case, merely taking a food break—may lead a judge to rule differently in cases with similar legal characteristics." Awareness of the findings of the study opens up space for self-correction in the interests of equal application of law.

Invisible and extra-legal factors at play

The impact of the visual impression on the psyche is another illustration of how invisible factors perhaps influence legal proceedings. *In the unfolding of the trial of cases under the anti-terrorism legislations and offences like sedition often couched in nebulous phrases, one can see the impact of the appearance of an accused who likely fits into the very picture in the mind of the judge of a "terrorist" of "anarchist" or "revolutionary" on the proceedings. Shukla (2011)* observes, "The category of 'hardcore Naxalite' is unknown to law. Yet the prosecution use and at every opportunity repeat, as in the case of Sen, that the accused associated with 'hardcore Naxalites'". The use is deliberate in terms of trying to cause prejudice in the mind of the judge" (p. 348).

Of gut feelings

There is widespread belief in the accuracy of "gut feelings." Stories of gamblers losing millions trusting their instinct are a legion. Perhaps, training in disciplines like research methodology, law, psychology, logic and science equips us to have accurate, dependable gut feelings which can be acted upon. Tversky and Kahneman (1971) call it the "gambler's fallacy" (p. 24) and on the basis of their research on and examination of psychological studies observe, "There were no differences in the median responses of audiences at a mathematical psychology meeting and at a general session of the American Psychological Convention, although we make no claims as to the representativeness of either sample. *Apparently, acquaintance with formal logic and with probability theory does not extinguish erroneous intuitions"* (pp. 29–30) (emphasis added). Paraphrasing Tversky and Kahenman, it is likely that "Apparently, knowledge and training in law does not extinguish erroneous intuitions."

Across the spectrum from the trial of an individual accused, to adjudicating the constitutionality of the anti-terror laws, the conscious and unconscious fantasies of judges of being "brave" little soldiers and protecting the mother and motherland and save her from dismemberment impact decision-making. In an unusual move, the first two paragraphs of the judgment of the Delhi High Court on interim bail in the case of Kanhaiya Kumar, the president of the Jawaharlal Nehru University Students Union, are comprised of stanzas of a patriotic song from the Hindi film "Upkaar" mentioned in paragraph two and excerpted below:

> *"1. 'Rang hara Hari Singh Nalve se, Rang laal hai Lal Bahadur se, Rang bana basanti Bhagat Singh, Rang aman ka veer Jawahar se.*
>
> *Mere Desh ki Dharti sona ugle Ugle here moti mere desh ki dharti'*
>
> *(Trans. The color green is from Hari Singh Nalve (a brave Sikh warrior), the color red is from Lal (meaning Red) from Lal Bahadur (the reference is to the second Prime Minister of India Lal Bahadur Shastri), the color saffron is form Bhagat Singh (martyr executed by the British in 1931), the color of peace from the brave Jawahar (the reference is to Jawahar Lal Nehru, the first Prime Minister of Independent India).*
>
> ("The earth of my land is gold and spews forth diamonds and pearls").
>
> 2. This patriotic song from 'Upkaar' by Lyricist Indeevar symbolizes individual characteristics representing by different colours and love for motherland."

Judgments of courts are generally couched in terms of fundamental rights of life and liberty and permissible reasonable restrictions and it is rare to find the subterranean factors at play explicitly articulated. Paragraph 41 of the judgment gives a fair idea of the role of the notions of "patriotism" at play in the rational and the logical arena of the law.

Paragraph 41:

> Suffice it to note that such persons enjoy the freedom to raise such slogans in the comfort of University Campus but without realizing that they are in this safe environment because our forces are there at the battle field situated at the highest altitude of the world where even the oxygen is so scarce that those who are shouting anti-national slogans holding posters of Afzal Guru and Maqbool Bhatt close to their chest honouring their martyrdom, may not be even able to withstand those conditions for an hour even.

Shukla (2017) observes "We find love for mother and motherland, anxiety of partition, the inimical attacking 'terrorists', the brave son protecting mother/motherland and the amputating-castrating mother all playing out in the Kanhaiya bail judgment" (p. 3). Baccheta (2004) writing of the depiction of motherland by ultra-nationalist organizations notes, "The Sangh presents her as a chaste mother, victimised (by Muslims) and declares that she needs the protection of her 'virile' sons, the 'Men with the capital M'. Unlike Kali, Bharatmata is left with no warrior qualities of her own" (p. 27).

Of national security, fears and offences

Statutes defining offences are as a rule precise, as they involve liberty of an individual and may lead to imprisonment. The run of the mill offences like "theft" and "cheating" clearly mentions the ingredients that have to be fulfilled to establish the commission of an offence. Laws with regard to national securities, perhaps reflecting anxieties about attack, encirclement and dismemberment, cast the net very wide. The provisions defining the offences are inevitably vague and wooly leaving much room for arbitrary use and the play of subjective notions of the Executive as well as the Judiciary. A case in point is the definition of sedition as "attempts or excites disaffection" towards the government. Disaffection literally means absence or alienation. The definition seems designed to give ample space to the ruling regimen of the day to detain any and everyone critical of the government of the day.

The anti-terrorism laws enacted over the decades are cast in the same mould as sedition. Thus, the Terrorist and Disruptive Activities (Prevention) Act, 1985; the Prevention of Terrorism Act, 2002 and the Unlawful Activities (Prevention) Act, 1967 all define offences like "terrorism," "disruptive activities" and "unlawful activities" in broad and imprecise terms. The vague definitions have led to the provisions being used against peaceful protests by farmers, agitations by workers or led to the targeting of minorities. Given the prevalence of the use of "third-degree" methods, euphemism for torture, confession to a police officer is not admissible as evidence in a court of law. However, this salutary provision has been given a go-by in the anti-terror laws and confession to a police officer has been declared to be admissible as evidence. The investigating agencies tend to use the easier path and often tailor and frame ordinary offences and charge the individuals under the more stringent anti-terror laws. Akin to the anti-drug laws, bail is near impossible but the concomitant speedy trial does not take place leading to periods of detention at times equal to the punishment provided for the offence in the statute.

Of vices, sex, sin and drugs

Akin to an invisible backstage influencer, the draughtsman plays a crucial role in the framing of the legislation upon which the edifice of law stands. Societal notions of vice, sin and immorality internalized in the draughtsman seems to play an all-pervasive role in the codifying of laws.

Suppression of Immoral Traffic Act to Immoral Traffic (Prevention) Act: SITA > IPTA

The very title of the legislation enacted in 1956 dealing with sex work in India was titled Suppression of Immoral Traffic Act – which translates into the acronym "SITA." The character "Sita" in the Hindu epic Ramayana is the very epitome of purity. The acronym SITA in capitals seems to point to the undeniable role of the notion of the pure virtuous woman and the sinful, immoral sex worker, aptly encapsulated by the phrase the "Whore and the Goddess," which seems the leitmotif of the statute. The nomenclature of the statute was changed into Immoral Traffic (Prevention) Act in 1986 and the acronym now stands as ITPA.

This law aimed at curbing human trafficking, criminalizes consenting adult sex workers under the guise of "rescue" of the woman from the pit of sin and immorality. In law, a crucial distinction is observed between an "adult" and a "minor." An adult has agency and is competent to give consent. A minor is deemed incompetent to give consent and the State is looked upon as the ultimate guardian of the minor. However, under ITPA, an adult with consent doing sex work can be "rescued" against their will. The police conduct a raid and detain the adult and in law, the person is categorized as "rescued." An accused person under the law can apply and be released on bail. However, the "rescued" person can be sent to a reform home for their moral betterment and does not have the provision to be released on bail. The moral thrust of the law makes a mockery of the fundamental right to life and liberty of the adult sex worker enshrined and guaranteed by the Constitution of India.

Of decoy customers

The statutes governing criminal procedure find no mention of the use of "decoy customers" as part of ploys authorized by law as legitimate methods for the collection of evidence to establish the commission of an offence. The Indian police are acutely overworked, yet vast number of resources are spent in the stratagem and deployment of "decoy customers" in the two arenas: sex work and narcotic substances. Elaborate operations are set up with "decoy customers" with marked notes sent to sex workers and to buy "drugs." The stratagem seems like an instigation to commit an offence and "entrapment" impermissible in law. In fact, it is difficult to imagine the police offering money to burgle a house and then catching the individual who takes up the offer and attempts it or that courts would accept such evidence. Perhaps, it points to the association with sin and vices that these methods are acceptable to establish the commission of offences in these "immoral" category of crimes.

Of presumption of guilt and indefinite detention

The presumption of innocence with the burden of proof being on the prosecution to establish an offence has been committed is sacrosanct in criminal law as it leads to curtailment of liberty. The Narcotics and Psychotropic Substances (Prevention of Abuse) Act, 1986 in a shocking departure from constitutional principles and criminal jurisprudence places the burden of proof on the accused to prove their innocence. It is likely that notions of and presumed linkages of sin, morality, vices, depravities, drugs, addictions and crime played a role in this dramatic reversal of a fundamental principle of law. The provisions of the statute make release on bail near impossible, premised on the promise of speedy trial and a swift conclusion to the proceedings. Instead, cases in courts are notoriously delayed, leading to years of incarceration with no prospect of release while awaiting trial.

Of social malaise statutes

Law attempts to fix social ills plaguing society have spawned a series of legislations. A look at the social legislation statutes proves to be instructive.

Anti-dowry legislation

The Dowry Prohibition Act, 1961 was brought in with the lofty objective of curbing the social evil of dowry and ushering in a society where marriages are not based on financial transactions and women are treated with respect and dignity. Dowry is the practice of giving of monies, movable property like cars and televisions or immovable property like houses and valuable security. Dowry is rampant and has wide societal acceptance in almost all religious communities. In workshops with judges to "Minimize the impact of biases, prejudices and stereotypes," the issue of dowry has been met with politically correct responses. Listening to response decrying dowry as a social evil, I am aware that after selection in the judicial service, the "market rate" would have gone up and bridegroom-to-be judges would command and receive a higher amount as dowry.

However, the acceptance and bias in favour of dowry of the drafters of the law is reflected in the provisions of the statute. The law makes the "giving" and "taking "of dowry an offence punishable with a minimum of five years imprisonment and a fine of 15,000 rupees. In the dynamics at play – the bride's family is coerced into giving dowry, and after marriage the now "wife" is ill-treated and abused to extract more dowry. In this context, equating the two parties and making the dowry giver liable for punishment ensured the death-knell of the anti-dowry law. There are hardly any convictions and the practice has enmeshed with consumerism and from being located in Hindu family practices has spread to other communities.

Law against sex-selective abortion

The sex ratio of the number of males to the number of females at birth is skewed in India, with fewer females born than males. The advance of technology leading to easy sex determination of the sex of the foetus through an ultra sound meshed in with the preference for "sons" who would get dowry over "daughter" who were burdens and dowry would have to be given in their marriages. The determination of the sex of the foetus was followed by the selective termination of pregnancy in case of the female foetus. Long and sustained campaign by the women's movement led to the enactment of the Pre-Natal Diagnostic Techniques (Prevention of Misuse) Act, 1994.

The law has been brought in for the laudable objective of the prohibition of sex selection, before or after conception and for the prevention of the misuse of pre-natal diagnostic techniques for sex determination leading to female foeticide. The technology is to be used only for detecting genetic abnormalities or metabolic disorders or chromosomal abnormalities. In tune with large-scale societal acceptance of sex selective abortion, the provisions of the law drafted make prosecutions near impossible. Perhaps, in tune with the prevalent social norms, the drafters consciously and/or unconsciously have made a married woman pressurized by her husband and in-laws to undergo the sex selection of the foetus and thereafter selective abortion in case of female foetus would be liable for punishment of three years and fine of 50,000 rupees. In order to escape punishment, the woman has to establish that she was "compelled to undergo such diagnostic techniques or such sex selection."[4] The provision making the victim woman liable in the context of the psychological and the socio-economic factors at play seems designed to ensure the failure of the law.

Of caste and law

Ironically, the impact of the unconscious with regard to caste is best illustrated in the working of the anti-caste laws in India. Caste is a pernicious feature of Indian society, which strikes at the roots of equality. Unlike natural disasters or wars where the trauma is linked to an event, the caste operates as inter-generational continuum across centuries. Koiliri (2025) speaking of the transmission of inter-generational trauma observes, "Collective trauma is when psychological trauma experienced by communities and identity groups is carried on as part of the group's collective memory and shared sense of identity." The Varna system of traditional Hindu thought visualized a pyramidal structure with the priestly Brahmins originating from the head at the top, Kshatriyas comprised of Kings and warriors from the arms, Vaishyas the traders and merchants from the thighs and Shudras working as unskilled workers from the feet. The untouchables were considered outside the Varna system and considered outcastes dealing with human and animal waste and dead bodies. Article 17 of the Constitution of India abolishes untouchability and forbids the practice making it punishable[5]. The practice flourishes and in fact, the caste system cuts across religions.

The two premier legislations in the field are the Untouchability Offences Act, 1955 rechristened in 1976 as the Protection of Civil Rights Act, 1955 (PCRA) and the SC/ST (Prevention of Atrocities) Act, 1989. Judges trying cases under the two legislations are alert to the nature of the cases and are consciously trying their best to be impartial. A look at the judgments points to the unconscious play of the upper-caste bias of the individuals on the bench. Given the miniscule representation of about 2.4% SC/ST persons in the higher judiciary reported by the National Commission of Schedule Castes (2011), it is likely that there will be more affinities between the caste of the judge and the accused with the complainant-victim being from a lower caste. We find that even though the provisions of law are clear, the judgments reflect an interpretation of law which works towards acquittal of the upper caste accused.

Caste abuses are often hurled in quarrels, the roots of which lie in the caste of the two parties. Yet, the courts have held that even though the accused flung a caste abuse, the offence would not fall within the ambit of the offence as there were other issues between the parties. The judgment of the Madhya Pradesh High Court declares, "On the other hand, if (the) insult had taken place only because the victim was a member of scheduled caste, and it would not have taken place if he had been of higher caste, then (the) insult was (an) insult on ground of untouchability." The Court goes on to cement the proposition, "Another rough and ready test, though not very infallible, would be to ask the question whether (the) insult was part of personal quarrel which took place between a person of higher caste and a member of the scheduled caste; or was the insult offered in (a) cool and studied manner in the absence of any quarrel. In the first situation, the insult would most likely (be) insult 'simpliciter' while in the second situation it would be (an) insult on the ground of untouchability".[6] Similarly, judges have worked around the provisions making distinctions between the insult being made in a "private" and not a "public" space[7] or seizing on the absence of the complainant, even though the caste insult was hurled at in a public place.[8]

The only instance of a sitting judge of a high court being sent to jail is of Justice Karnan, a Dalit judge. The genesis of the events started from a complaint from Justice Karnan that the upper-caste judge sitting cross-legged next to him deliberately touched him with his shoe, then said sorry and two other judges were watching and smiling. Justice Karnan also complained that he was discriminated against on the basis of caste at several get-togethers such as full court meetings, high tea and dinner. The matter escalated and finally ended with the conviction for contempt of court and incarceration of Justice Karnan.[9]

Of judges and working of laws

> Reflecting on this case we feel convinced that a socially sensitized judge is a better statutory armour against gender outrage than long clauses of a complex section with all the protections writ into it.

Justice Krishna Iyer

The Supreme Court of India acquitted two policemen convicted of custodial rape in 1977.[10] The case, referred to as the 'Mathura rape case', led to huge protests by the women's movement and respected academics. This resulted in change in the law of evidence in 1983 introducing a provision stating that if a woman states that she did not consent to sexual intercourse, the court shall presume that she did not consent.[11] Similarly, an amendment to the law, which came into force in 2003, categorically laid down that "Provided that in a prosecution for rape or attempt to commit rape, it shall not be permissible to put questions in the cross-examination of the prosecutrix as to her general immoral character."[12] The amendment omitted the corresponding provision[13] permitting impeaching of the character of the woman from the Indian Evidence Act, 1872.

The impact of entrenched attitudes of judges comes through in judgments in cases of rape, despite the clear words of the new provision with regard to presumption of lack of consent. Even after the two amendments in law submissions, such as "the prosecutrix was examined by Doctor A. The doctor found no injuries on any parts of her body including to her private parts," still weigh with the courts in acquitting or convicting the accused of rape. In the face of the statute placing a total bar on impeaching the credit of the witness, the courts continue to declare in judgments "It must however be conceded that immoral character would still not be an absolutely irrelevant circumstance. It may render the story itself as incredible. It may take away probative force of the story, told as it is by a woman with no scruples or morals."[14]

In fact, we can see the crucial role that the psyche of the judge plays in the arena of criminal too. The working of the Rajasthan Sati (Prevention) Act, 1987 in courts is a case in point. The statute lays down the definition: *"Sati" means the burying or buying alive of any widow along with the body of her deceased husband or with any article, object or thing associated with the husband, irrespective of whether such burning or burying is voluntary on the part of the widow or otherwise:*[15] "Glorification of sati is defined as *'glorification' in relation to Sati, includes among other things, the observance of any ceremony or the taking out of a procession in connection with Sati or the creation of a trust or the collection of funds or the construction of a temple or the performance of any ceremony thereat with a view to perpetuating the honour of, or to preserve the memory of, a widow committing Sati."*[16] The Additional District and Sessions Judge, Neem-ka-thana in Rajasthan, acquitted all the accused of the charges of Sati and Sati glorification and declared sati as a "woman being virtuous, having strong character, completely devoted towards her husband and having a relationship with only one man during her whole life." Applying this interpretation, the judgment refers to Sita and Anusuya as satis and observes that the invocation of their name would obviously not make a person guilty of sati glorification.

The mindset of the judge impacts cases under ordinary criminal law under the Indian Penal Code, 1875. Bhanwari Devi was a village level working for the prevention of child marriages prevalent in Rajasthan. She has successfully prevented the child marriage of the daughter of one of the accused persons. On 22 September 1992, she was gang-raped by five men who were accused of the heinous offence. Shukla (2006) observes, "According to the judge, the accused are middle aged and therefore respectable citizens, while teenagers usually commit rape. The judgment goes on to declare, "Since the accused are upper-caste men, the rape could not have taken place because Bhanwari was from a lower caste."

Of Justice as divine or judges as mortals

> A faithful God who does no wrong, upright and just is He.
> (Deuteronomy 32:4)

Song of Moses

> According to him, human justice was nothing and divine justice was everything. I pointed out it was the former that had condemned me.
> *Albert Camus, The Stranger*

Healy (1950) in his review, "Courts on Trial, Myths and Reality in American Justice" by Justice Jerome Frank observes that – The virile chapter on 'The Cult of the Robe' shows what Judge Frank is after, namely, to have an intelligent public understand 'that the springs of decision in judges' do not 'differ from the springs of decision in other men'. The wearing of the robe and legal jargon tend to becloud that fact."

People litigate and come to courts with wrongs, grievances, conflicts and disputes. Judges have to manage the emotions of a plethora of people's distraught victims, witnesses, the adversary parties and the perpetrators. At times, judges have to cajole, reprimand, cool temperatures and keep the discourse in courts civilized. Irritation at the pomp and show – the robes, the "all rise" in court at the entry of the judge, the close to genuflecting to the judicial chair, the "your lordship," "your honour" peppering any submission – has given way to a grudging recognition that the quaint formal practices to maintain decorum perhaps play a crucial role in containing emotions at play in courtrooms. Leaving the area of matrimonial disputes and child custody battles which seem to bring out particularly volatile emotions for engagement later, we move on to the one crucial area which seems universally unaddressed by legal systems the emotions of judges.

The judge as an absolute creature of rationality and reason – a modern-day Solomon – seems to be the conception underpinning the legal system. Lalit, J. (2022), a judge of the Supreme Court of India, who went on to become the next Chief Justice of India, observed "When you're arguing as a counsel, you argue purely on facts and law, allowing emotions to be kept out." Perhaps, the story of Solomon the wise from the bible[17] has pointers to the complex play of emotions and logic in the process and is worth a recap. Two women were claiming a child. Solomon ordered the child cut in half. The woman who pleaded that the child be given to the other woman was declared to be the mother.

As we cut to ground realities of courtrooms and judges in India – we come to the Priyadarshini Mattoo case. Priyadarshini, a third-year law student, was found strangled to death in her bedroom in Delhi on 23 January 1996 with 19 injuries on her person. Santosh Kumar Singh, a law student and son of a senior officer of the Indian Police Service the accused, was acquitted of the charge of rape and murder. The declaration by the Additional Sessions Judge, Delhi G. P. Thareja: "Though I know he is the man who committed the crime, I acquit him, giving him the benefit of doubt" is a pointer to the frustrations of a judge's life in India. The accused being the son of a senior police officer is likely to have played a role in lax investigation by the police.

In the hierarchy of the judiciary, the constitutional courts like high courts and the Supreme Court exercise appellate jurisdiction and original jurisdiction in case of violation of fundamental rights and certain specified areas like inter-state disputes or petitions to transfer a case from one to another. These courts function in a rarefied atmosphere far from the hurly-burly of life. Sitting on throne like chairs the judges are addressed by medieval phrases like "Milord" or "Your Lordship", used to refer to English noblemen and quaint submissions like "I bow to what has fallen from your Lordship's lips." The higher courts have negligible interface with ordinary people and interact with sophisticated lawyers.

Thumbnail sketch of a trial court in India

It is sessions judges like Mr. Thareja who try serious offences like murder and rape and the magistrates who deal with lesser offences who are the backbone of the legal system. They function among abysmal conditions. The scorching Indian summer with a whirring ceiling fan throwing out hot air in the courtroom among the broken down chairs, littered dirty corridors and leaking toilets are the setting for lower courts. The workload of judges is unimaginable – 150 cases may be fixed before a single judge on a day. Tempers are on a short fuse in the heat and in addition to dealing with highly strung aggrieved parties, judges have to contain and manage aggressive lawyers in a slanging match. The police, who seem to wield unchecked power in India, chafe at the constraints to behave civilly in court premises and judges at times have to deal with lawyer-police skirmishes.

Akin to Sessions Judge Thareja who despite being sure of the guilt was constrained to acquit the accused son of a high ranking police officer due to lacunae in investigation, Magistrates and Judges are confronted everyday by parties and witnesses who are clearly lying, or corrupt policemen who have been bribed and have deliberately fudged data and investigation, leading to engendering utter frustration. In contrast to the logo of the judiciary "*Satyamev Jayate*" – "Truth alone Triumphs," apocryphal stories circulating in courts are pointers to the utter cynicism which judges encounter daily in the course of their work. An accused requests his lawyer to not keep the day of his testimony in court on Tuesdays. Query reveals that on account of the observance of a religious fast, the accused does not lie on Tuesdays. A pickpocket being tried for the offence after the hearing requests his lawyer for an hour's time to pay his fees. The accused goes around the crowded courts, picks pockets and returns within the hour and hands over the fee to his counsel. The helplessness of being a mere cog in the wheel that sees injustice being perpetuated in his own courtroom permeates the existence of a judicial officer. After an exhausting time, at the end of the day, a magistrate going home may find himself travelling in the same crowded public transport as the accused. The judgments of trial courts are considered too insignificant and are not reported in journals and there are no studies like the Australian interviews of magistrates.

Anleu and Mack (2005) interviewed 46 Magistrates (29 men and 17 women) in every state in Australia from the standpoint of emotional labour as these are the interface of the judiciary with the people and offer certain vignettes that convey the texture of the life of a trial court judicial officer in any legal system. Thereafter, a National Survey of Australian Magistrates in Australia showed: "Thus, a total of two in three magistrates (66 per cent) consider managing the emotions of court users to be at least a very important skill" (p. 606).

A Magistrate articulates the experience "You're seeing absolute misery passing in front of you day in, day out, month in, month out, year in, year out; you're seeing women with young kids having to go to gaol, you're seeing young ... all of this misery, day in, day out" (p. 611). Another Magistrate articulates the impact of the experience "Now, there's two things that can happen to you. Either you're going to remain a decent person and become terribly upset by it all because your emotions because your feelings are being pricked by all of this constantly or you're going to become - you're going to grow a skin on you as thick as a rhino, in which case I believe you're going to become an inadequate judicial officer because once you lose the human - the feeling for humanity you can't really I don't believe you can do the job" (p. 612).

Family courts deal with tremendous resentments and antagonisms generated in intimate relationships and a Magistrate evocatively puts it in words "....... I've heard about families and the stress that they're under, the treatment children have been dished out, what will happen to them for the rest of their lives. I just find it difficult to walk away from that and go home to my own children and look at them and think 'Oh, God', you know. .... So it's just the sadness; there is no good news" (p. 613).

Perhaps, the agonies and frustrations of judicial life cut across countries and we find Pregerson J. (dissenting) 2007, a judge in the United States, observing "Sometimes [the judge] has to just sit up there and watch justice fail right in front of him, right in his own courtroom, and he doesn't know what to do about it, and it makes him feel sad.... Sometimes he even gets angry about it."[18]

Of the head and the heart

> The law, in its majestic equality, forbids rich and poor alike to sleep under bridges, to beg in the streets, and to steal their bread.

Anatole France (1894)

Judges as implacable beings dispensing justice inexorably is the dominant imago that rules the legal system. In contrast to a dialectical interplay, law seems to carry the conflict of the head and the heart which we may at times feel in life to an extreme. Solomon's two-mother story seems to be a neat illustration of the role of both reason and emotion.

In the context of the rational versus emotional paradigm, Kakar (2008) writes "A complex mind will be guided by both the visions, the romantic enlivening and lending a 'poetic' sensibility and sentiment to reason while the rational vision guards against the sentimental excesses to which the romantic is all too susceptible" (p. 3). Maroney (2011) observes "In contrast to the Enlightenment view that emotion and reason are at war, contemporary theorists are forging a new consensus that emotion is a necessary element of much of the practical and moral reasoning on which law depends" (p. 648). Maroney goes on to posit "Emotion's critical role in reflecting and enabling reason coexists with an ability to shape our experience and expression of it in accordance with a hierarchy of reasons" (p. 649). Jackson J. (1944), an American judge, in contrast to the ponderous language associated with law. points out that "dispassionate judges" are "mythical beings" like "Santa Claus or Uncle Sam or Easter bunnies."

Of the way forward

The first interface of the citizen is the police performing a vital component in the criminal-correctional process. Rathod (2026), a psychologist-researcher emphasizing the long work hours, the exposure to trauma leading to Post-Traumatic Stress Disorder (PTSD), Anxiety, Depression and a work culture where admitting to emotional struggles is perceived as weakness with stigma, reports, "According to a 2017 survey conducted by the Bureau of Police Research and Development (BPRD), a significant number of police officers admitted to using alcohol and other substances as a coping mechanism for job-related stress. The survey indicated that about 34% of officers consumed alcohol frequently, with a notable portion reporting dependency issues. Anecdotal evidence and regional studies highlight the use of illegal substances, though comprehensive national data remains sparse." The ambit of the present work is the exploration of the world of the judge, the dispenser of justice. However, it is no less important to chart the world of the police and acknowledge the high stress nature of the work and set up support structures and services to assist in dealing with anxieties, depression, PTSD and substance abuse.

At present, the terrain of the emotional forms no part in the training of a judge. A judicial officer has to take on board his/her own emotions, process and contain them, an enterprise which is daunting enough. In a double whammy, unlike the relatively insulated appellate courts, a trial court judge has to deal with raging aggravating negative emotions of a wide variety of individuals – grieving parents, aggrieved spouses, distraught children, righteous prosecutors, aggressive lawyers – to mention a few. The role of a judge demands an unflappable calm demeanour. The tremendous stress and effort put in – the invisible "emotional labour" is not taken on board by the legal system. The calm demeanour does not mean that the feelings evoked have magically vanished.

A first step of a formal acknowledgement by the legal system of emotional labour as an important component of the function as a judge would validate the feelings rather than the emotions, anxieties and fears evoked in the individual feeding into feelings of inadequacy as a judge. Access and availability of individual therapy sessions should be made available as a matter of routine and not come with the stigma of a "judge who could not cope with the pressures" or being offered it as charity or concession. Rather than top-down approach of diktats by superior courts, it is the trial court judges and magistrates who are the best judges of what would work and their involvement is crucial in evolving group processes towards less stressful existence and a more fulfilling life, in turn contributing to the health of the legal system in India.

Notes

1 The Supreme Court of India approvingly quoted the phrase in the 1978 case titled Madhav Hayawadanrao Hoskote versus State of Maharashtra.
2 Swami Vivekananda, The Yogas and Other Works, ed. S. Nikbilananda, New York: Ramakrishna-Vivekananda Center, 1953, pp. 608–609.
3 As to the baggage carried in terms of biases, prejudices and stereotypes and the impact of extra-legal factors, please see the chapter titled "Inner World of Judges: Psychoanalytical Explorations."
4 Section 23(4) of the Pre-Natal Diagnostic Techniques (Prevention of Misuse) Act, 1994.
5 Article 17 of the Constitution of India. Abolition of untouchability. "Untouchability" is abolished and its practice in any form is forbidden. The enforcement of any disability arising out of "Untouchability" shall be an offence punishable in accordance with law. "Untouchability" is abolished and its practice in any form is forbidden. The enforcement of any disability arising out of "Untouchability" shall be an offence punishable in accordance with law.
6 Phulsing vs State of Madhya Pradesh 1991 Criminal Law Journal 2954.
7 2 'IDBI Chief Arrested for Caste Abuse', The Telegraph, 7 May 2005.
8 E Krishnan Nayanar vs Dr M A Kuttappan, Member Kerala Legislative Assembly and others, 1997 Criminal Law Journal 2036.
9 Further reading on the issue, please see: "To Remove Caste bias from the judicial system, Judges need to self-correct. Shukla (2017).
10 State of Maharashtra versus Tukaram.
11 Section 114 A of the Indian Evidence Act, 1872 introduced by the Criminal Law Amendment Act, 1983.
12 The Indian Evidence (Amendment) Act 2002 – No. 4 of 2003.
13 Clause 4 of Section 154 of the Indian Evidence Act, 1872 was omitted.
14 Banti Alias Balvinder Singh vs State Of Madhya Pradesh on 3 September 1991. https://indiankanoon.org/doc/413657/. Retrieved 1 September 2025.
15 Section 2(c) of the Rajasthan Sati (Prevention) Act, 1987.
16 Section 2(b) of the Rajasthan Sati (Prevention) Act, 1987.
17 Old Testament (1 Kings 3:16–28).
18 Carrington v. United States, 503 F.3d 888, 899 (9th Cir. 2007) (Pregerson, J., dissenting).

Bibliography

Anleu. S.R. and Mack K. 2005. Magistrates' Everyday Work and Emotional Labour. Journal of Law and Society, Vol. 32, No. 4 (Dec., 2005), pp. 590–614 Published by: Wiley on behalf of Cardiff University Stable URL: http://www.jstor.org/stable/3557252. Retrieved 5th September 2025.

Baccheta, P. 2004. Gender in the Hindu Nation, RSS Women as Ideologues. New Delhi: Women Unlimited (an associate of Kali for Women).

Brennan, Jr. W.J. 1972. Furman v. Georgia, 408 U.S. 238 (1972). Quoted by Supreme Court of India in Madhav Hayawadanrao Hoskot vs State of Maharashtra. 1978 All India Reporter 1548. https://indiankanoon.org/doc/513169/. Retrieved 08th August 2025.

Danziger. S, Leval J. and Avnaim-Pesso L. 2011. Extraneous factors in judicial decisions. https://www.pnas.org/doi/epdf/10.1073/pnas.1018033108. Retrieved 08th August 2025.

France, A. 1894. Le Lys rouge (The Red Lily). Chapter 7, pp. 111–123.

Freud, S. 1933. New Introductory Lectures on Psychoanalysis. Revised Standard Edition, Vol. 22, pp. 65–66.

Healy, W. 1950. Courts on trial. Myths and realities in American Justice by Jerome Frank. Review. Psychoanalytic Quarterly, Vol. 19, pp. 437–438.

Jackson, J. (dissenting). 1944. Unites States v. Ballard, 322 U.S. 78, 93–94 (1944).

Kakar, S. 1981. The Inner World, A Psychoanalytical Study of Childhood and Society in India. Oxford University Press. New Delhi.

Kakar, S. 2008. Mad and Divine, Spirit and Psyche in the Modern World. New Delhi: Penguin Viking.

Koiliri, A.K. 2025. Healing The Psyche from Caste Violence: Addressing the Cumulative Psychological Trauma of Generations of Oppression and Deprivation Among the SC/ST Community in India. The International Journal of Indian Psychology ISSN 2348-5396 (Online) | ISSN: 2349-3429 (Print) Volume 13, Issue 2, April- June, 2025. DIP: 18.01.125.20251302, DOI: 10.25215/1302.125. https://ijip.in/wp-content/uploads/2025/05/18.01.125.20251302.pdf. Retrieved 29th August 2025.

Lalit, U.U. 2022. in Ojha, S. 'Argue on facts and law, avoid emotions': What SC Judge told lawyers'. https://www.indiatoday.in/law/story/argue-on-facts-law-emotions-to-be-avoided-sc-judge-uu-lalit-1981678-2022-07-30. Retrieved 5th September 2025.

Maroney, T.A. 2011. The persistent script of Judicial Dispassion. California Law Review. Vol. 99(2), pp. 629–681.

National Commission of Schedule Castes. 2011. A Report on Reservation in Judiciary. https://ncsc.nic.in/storage/special_events/owpsaxblMRcpFAU0XZaRNTaFxkyG1DI3jEEYt3gX.pdf. Retrieved 28th August 2025.

(Pregerson, J., dissenting). 2007. Carrington v. United States, 503 F.3d 888, 899 (9th Cir. 2007).

Rathod, Rajnandini. 2026. The impact of substance abuse on law enforcement in India. https://rehabs.in/news/impact-of-substance-abuse-on-law-enforcement-officers-in-india/. Retrieved 22nd January 2026.

Shukla, R. 2006. Judiciary and Caste. Economic and Political Weekly, October 21, 2006.

Shukla, R. 2011. Judging Sedition: The Case of the Good Doctor. International Journal of Applied Psychoanalytic Studies. Studies, Vol. 8(4), pp. 346–352.

Shukla, R. 2017a. "To Remove Caste bias from the judicial system, Judges need to self-correct". thewire.in/caste/caste-bias-judicial-system. Retrieved 28th August 2025.

Shukla, R. 2017b. Mother, Motherland and the Judicial Function: the Case of Kanhaiya Kumar. International Journal of Applied Psychoanalytic Studies, Vol. 14, pp. 305–307.

Shukla, R. 2019. Quest for justice: Psychoanalytical explorations with judges. In Plinio M. & Harris A. (eds) Psychoanalysis, Law and Society. Routledge. London.

Tversky, A., & Kahneman, D. 1971. Belief in the Law of Small Numbers. Psychological Bulletin, 76, pp. 105–110.

Venkatesh, N.A. 2024. The Need for Empathic Judging. The India Forum. https://www.theindiaforum.in/law/need-empathic-judging. Retrieved 18th September, 2025.

4 Trauma and Testimony

Memory, the Psyche and the Demands of Law

Judge: *How far were you from the place of occurrence?*
Witness: *21 meters, 53 centimeters Mi'lord!*
Judge: *How come you are so precise?*
Witness: *I measured it Mi'lord! I knew some fool would ask me.*

The joke doing the round in the corridors of courts does illustrate in a lighter vein the demands of testimony in law from the survivor-victims of violent events.

Law in all its majesty demands a linear narration of events, logical consistency, a clear time line and a precision of corroborative detail of the facts and circumstances surrounding the occurrence. Coherence, which is the individual's ability to give answers that address the questions, put to the witness and which can be understood individually and collectively is a crucial component of credible testimony in law. Unfortunately, the impact of trauma on the psyche induces a state of mind, which makes it very difficult to satisfy the precision of corroborative detail requirements of law. The occurrence of an event perceived as threatening to well-being and existence activates the threat detector parts of the brain, releases adrenaline and may induce panic attacks, terror, an urge to flee or may cause a freeze and shut down.

A fragmentation occurs wherein memory is stored in sensory fragments of smells, sounds and visuals, which is not verbally accessible memory. Brewin et al. make a distinction between a person's conscious experience of the trauma, which they categorize as accessible knowledge that can be retrieved and term it "verbally accessible memory (VAMs)" (p. 676) and flashbacks. They posit a parallel second set of memories and write, "The output of the more extensive nonconscious processing of the traumatic situation will form a second set of representation or set of representations that cannot be deliberately accessed. Brewin (1989) termed this situationally accessible knowledge because the representations may be accessed automatically when the person is in a context in which the physical features or meaning are similar to those of the

DOI: 10.4324/9781003626794-5

traumatic situation." Like a dialogue in a play, a scene in a movie or a recounting of a story may suddenly bring the memory to the fore.

Trauma may cause the blurring of timelines, events and places and at times a mixing up of stories of several different people, more so in incidents of collective violence and trauma. Traumatic memories may tend to be fragmented and internally inconsistent rather than a cohesive smoothly flowing narrative. Trauma may make a person hypervigilant and fidgety and in a courtroom may be perceived as a nervous and jittery witness raising suspicions about the reliability of the testimony. On the other hand, a mother whose child had been murdered may be deposing and describing the events in a flat monotone, as the emotional detachment may be helping her in coping with the distress, but may be perceived by the judge as lacking affect and not in tune with the ordinary course of human nature, and perhaps, looked upon as not such a credible witness.

At present, there is no psycho-emotional component in the training of judges to sensitize them to see where the trauma survivors are "coming from" to use an informal but evocative phrase. There is little space for an understanding of the impact of trauma on the psyche, the emotional state and the psycho-social matrix of the trauma survivor. Trauma survivors cut a sorry figure in courts in the adversarial criminal justice system with cross-examinations designed to destabilize and shake their testimony as witnesses. In the anti-Muslim pogram of 2002 in the Gujarat state of India, Zaheera Sheikh, a 19-year-old woman, witnessed the killing of 11 members of her family and three Hindu employees and the setting of fire to the Best Bakery run by her family in the city of Baroda. Zaheera was the crucial witness and the complainant in the criminal complaint against the accused persons. In a textbook illustration of insensitivity, the legal system did little to protect the young woman from the pressures, which may have been brought to bear, which lead her to change the testimony. The Supreme Court of India convicted Zaheera Sheikh for contempt of court and sentenced her to one-year's imprisonment and Rs. 50,000 fine to be paid within two months and in case of default, a further imprisonment of one year in the case of Zahira Habibullah Sheikh (2006).[1] The attitude of the court can be gauged from the fact that the maximum punishment for contempt of court is six months imprisonment.[2]

Shukla (2015) observes "The harsh dynamics of repeated depositions and cross examinations end up showing the victim–survivor as inconsistent, contradictory and lacking credibility. In a number of cases, rather than taking on board the vulnerabilities and pressures working on the victim–survivor, the system may end up further victimizing the victim–survivor. In the worst case scenario the trauma survivor who has suffered violence or been witness to brutal killing and rape is shown to have lied on oath leading to prosecution and imprisonment for perjury."

Psycho-social matrix

Like in the Best Bakery Zahira case of mass violence targeting the Muslim community in 2002 or the 1984 killing of Sikhs, the perpetrators are from sections of society with significant political power and influence in the police bureaucracy. Similar is the matrix in the series of killings by landlords and upper-caste men of historically oppressed so-called 'lower' castes, especially the hitherto untouchable castes.[3] The genesis of individual crimes often lies in the same socio-economic matrix. The first step of approaching the appropriate authorities to make a complaint is itself a herculean task fraught with pitfalls. There is a lurking fear that making the complaint may lead to retaliation, which may worsen the situation for the vulnerable community and the individual witness-survivor. Even after mustering up courage and taking the step, there are valid fears that the police might not register the complaint. In cases of sexual violence at an internal level, there may be feelings of self-blame, perhaps they provoked the perpetrator. That nobody will believe or listen to them accompanied by feelings of helplessness and isolation of the survivor-victim. There may be apprehensions that the family will blame them along with feelings of having brought shame to the family, which further compound the stressful situation, making it difficult to take steps with an immediacy demanded by law. Delay in reporting by the survivor inevitably works in favour of the accused-perpetrator. Talwar (2024) based on her extensive doctoral study of interventions and support for adult Child Sexual Abuse (CSA) survivors notes, "They were uncertain of their families', especially parents', reactions. Participants feared that they would not be believed and would be dismissed or blamed. Some of the survivors wondered if they would burden or risk hurting their loved ones by informing them that the survivors have been exploited" (p. 177).

Trauma impact

The present section looks at the effects of trauma on victim – survivors of sexual abuse including children and the functioning of the legal system.

Talwar (2024) in her doctoral thesis reports the findings, "Survivors' difficulties are likely to include low self-esteem, mood disturbances, anhedonia, irritability, self-blame, obsessions and compulsions, impulsivity, flashbacks, nightmares, suicidal ideas and intent (including deliberate self-harm). These difficulties may also include fears of revictimisation, decreased or increased interest in sexual activities, impulsivity, paranoia, difficulty concentrating, headaches and physical pain, sleep disturbances, problems in sense of self and safety, anger, shame and disgust" (p. 203). Padampriya and Alagesen (2024) through their case study in South India research the impact of sexual abuse on the physical and mental health of the survivors and emphasize the need for comprehensive support and observe, "Sexual harassment is the most distressing phenomenon, and in most situations, the victims are afraid of telling that they are the victims of sexual abuse due to the negative impacts they have to face in society. For instance, blaming the victim, isolating them, and making them homeless are such negative impacts that the survivor has to suffer along with their abuse. Healthcare providers need to provide extra care when handling CSA survivors, which can have positive impacts on their lives" (p. 4).

Roth et al (1997) conducted a study of post-traumatic stress disorder in victims exposed to sexual and physical abuse in 234 participants. The study had 189 women (81%) of the sample and 45 (19%) were men. Eighty-nine percent (207) of the sample were White, 9% (22) were Black and 2% (5) were Other. The study reports alterations in regulation of affect and impulses in the areas of Anger; Self-Destructive; Suicidal Preoccupation, Modulation of Sexual Involvement and Excessive Risk Taking. Amnesia; Transient Dissociative episodes and Depersonalization and feelings of Despair; Helplessness; Permanent Damage; Guilt and Responsibility; Shame; Inability to trust; Revictimization and Victimizing others were some other findings. Idealization of the perpetrator and Preoccupation with hurting the perpetrator are both possible impacts of the abuse. At a somatic level, it can lead to chronic back pain, headaches, nausea, diarrhoea and bloating, in addition to difficulties in the sexual domain, irregular menstruation and painful intercourse (p. 541).

Acknowledgement in law

The Indian legal system is little tuned to the state of the mind of the survivor-victim. Instead, legal processes seem to contribute substantially to the trauma of the survivor. The 84th Report of the Law Commission of India submitted in 1980 on "Rape and Allied Offences: Some Questions of Substantive Law, Procedure and Evidence" notes: "1.2 It is often stated that a woman who is raped undergoes two crises, the rape and the subsequent trial. While the first seriously moves her dignity, curbs her individual, disturbs her sense of security and may often ruin her physically, the second is no less potent of mixture, in as much as it not only forces her to relive through the traumatic experience, but also does so in the grudge of publicity in a totally alien atmosphere, with the whole apparatus and paraphernalia of the criminal justice system focused upon her." The Report of the Justice J.S. Verma (2013) Committee to amend criminal law formed after the brutal gang rape of a young woman in 2012,[4] chaired by ex-Chief Justice of India J.S. Verma with Justice Leila Seth and Shri Gopal Subramanium as members endorsed the observations of the 84th Law Commission Report on "Rape and Allied Offences: Some Questions of Substantive Law, Procedure and Evidence" and the recommendations eventually led to the Criminal Law Amendment Act, 2013. Shukla (2014) provides an analysis of the emotions like anger and fury, the protests, the police action and the processes at play.

Individual judges have at times acknowledged the impact of trauma and subsequent legal process on the psyche of the survivor. Justice Mittal (2009) in the Delhi High Court judgment while dealing with a case of child sexual abuse observes, "Children who are victims of sexual assaults and rape carry a huge burden of unwarranted guilt and violations for which they are not responsible. The humiliation, shame and embarrassment which cloud their emotions because of the worst kind of violation they have suffered which get aggravated when required to recount the same to strangers in formal surroundings. The trauma of a child victim is only multiplied as he or she is required to repeatedly recapitulate her ordeal to the investigating agencies, prosecutors and then in court" (p. 2744).

There is no single agreed upon definition of a vulnerable witness. Factors in the nature of being under the age of 17 years, suffering from mental disorder, impairment of intelligence and social functioning or physical disability, categorize an individual as vulnerable witness. An intimidated witness would be one whose quality of evidence is diminished by reason of fear or distress and would depend on the factors in the nature of the relation with the accused, social, cultural and economic background of the parties, the age of the person, the nature of complaint including whether it involves sexual offences. In case of vulnerable witnesses – special attunement and efforts are needed by the judge to create a comfort zone for the witness-survivor to be able to depose as to the traumatic events.

Role of the judge

The court is the domain of the judiciary. The judge anchors the proceedings and sets the atmosphere and tenor in the courtroom. The behaviour, the manner of address, the pitch and tone of the voice and the body language of the judge contribute to the level of comfort felt by a witness deposing in court. In case of vulnerable and intimidated witnesses, these factors assume an even greater role. The role of the judge is one as the very epitome of rationality and logic. In courts in India, the judges sit on an elevated throne like chair before which everyone stands and bows down upon arrival of the individual adorning the bench. The combination of representing rationality, logic and justice makes it particularly difficult for the judge to touch or access feelings of vulnerability and helplessness in one. On the other hand, if the judge could get in touch with emotions which the trauma survivor may be experiencing, it may be a vital factor, which would help in making the courtroom friendlier for deposition of a vulnerable witness. It would give cues for interventions that would contribute to the creation of a zone of comfort for the trauma survivor.

Trauma sensitization intervention in judicial training

Applying and taking the psychoanalytical perspective further[5] into the field of judicial training, I designed and conducted a two-part workshop at the Delhi Judicial Academy titled "Testimonies of trauma: Assisting judges understand troubled narratives."[6] Images and phrases were selected and projected onto a screen, with the object of evoking the feelings that perhaps are swamping and overwhelming the survivor-victim. The aim was as a first step for the judges to get in touch with and articulate the feelings triggered by the projections. This entailed each individual participant making efforts to get in touch with their emotions and as a second step their free associations, which were to be articulated as a second step of the workshop. In order to demonstrate the methodology of the workshop, specimen slides were projected and it was explained that in the first round, one was to get in touch with the feelings evoked and articulate them. A slide showing the picture of a disabled girl was projected evoking emotions like sympathy and pity. In the second round, associations and thoughts were to be expressed, for example, that there is a disability rights act; the person should explore possibilities of going to court to get her rights and go for medical treatment.

Some of the images projected were of a cowering frightened girl with dark shadows looming over her; line drawing of a distraught trapped figure behind bars in a cage-like structure; line drawing depicting a human figure with the thought bubble – "they are all talking about me"; a man fingers clenched, eyes open, hair standing, screaming in frustration; a slide on which it is written over and over again "why does this happen to me only'; a man hiding his face with his hands with many fingers pointing at him; two angry men with their foreheads against each other screaming; a human figure drawing with a trunk on the back with "Guilt Grade A" emblazoned on it; two forearms chained at the wrists. The last two images are of a lighthouse emitting a stream of light in the stormy seas and a little boy nurturing and watching a little plant grow. Some of the responses of the participants to a couple of images follow to illustrate the texture of the workshop methodology.

The emotions evoked in the participants by the image of frightened girl and the woman behind bars were Fear, Vulnerability, Anxiety, Helplessness, Frustration, Hearing voices, Feeling of being trapped, Creepy and the associations were Oversensitive, Self-hate, Lack of trust, Weird, Schizophrenia, Imaginations and Begging for life. The slide depicting the line figure with the thought bubble – "they are all talking about me" evoked feelings of Self-pity, Insecurity, Self-consciousness and Insecurity and the associations were Distorted Self-Image, Social Anxiety, Persecution, Societal violation and Negative. The angry screaming men images evoked Anger, Frustration, Aggression, Fear, Irritation, Disgust, Bitterness and the associations were Negative, Repulsiveness and Funny. The fingers pointing at man with face hidden behind hands evoked Humiliation, Sympathy, Shame, Guilt and the associations were putting the blame on me, I haven't done anything, Go away and Escape.

The creation of a comfort zone where the victim-survivor can depose freely is not something which can be achieved through myriad statutory provisions and rules. The setting and the function of the judge is one which makes it very difficult to get in touch with the universe of the victim-survivor witness. The delicate balance, the porcelain like fragility which can tip over at any moment into a meltdown or panic attack, is the world of the vulnerable witness. There is perhaps, a constant alertness and being on edge at possible lurking danger, harm and threat to one's existence. The judicial function requires a distancing from feelings of vulnerability and helplessness and likely the judge would find it difficult to get in touch with these feelings in themselves. If the individual sitting on the bench can for a fraction of a second experience some of the emotions evoked in the workshop while hearing the case, it may help in giving cues to create a space where the witness is able to depose freely. These could be in the areas of the conduct and appearance of the various actors in the court setting like directing that police personnel not to appear in uniform for deposing or when present in court. There could be telltale signs as to body language, tone and expressions, which in turn could guide an attuned court in modulating the proceedings. The court could direct breaks in the proceedings and fix smaller timelines from the usual schedule of hearings, direct the use of one-way mirror, screens, curtains or other devices.

Intra- and inter-psychic processes

Knowledge and familiarity with intra- and inter-psychic processes does not seem to be part of the training imparted to individuals to equip them to discharge the judicial role. The second part of the workshop took the same frame forward and briefly explained the processes and then facilitated the participants to think of instances from their own life where these processes may have been at play. The aim was for the judges to be able to see the processes at play in the testimony of trauma survivors with a perspective that does not categorize and stigmatize as conscious lies and deceit or attempts to mislead the court. That the defences and psychic processes were unconscious coping mechanisms to reduce anxiety, unacceptable impulses, painful areas and feelings as distinct from conscious coping mechanisms. Denial as if a painful event or feeling did not exist; regression or reversion to an earlier stage of development; acting out behaviour as expression of felt emotion instead of articulation; disassociation or disconnect with the thoughts, feelings and memories were all mechanisms to cope with unbearable traumatic events and feelings. These mechanisms manifesting in the testimony are not to be held against the witness and adverse inferences in law as to reliability and credibility drawn to the detriment of the trauma survivor. That painful events cause psychological damage and at times, a conflation of different incidents, dates, times and occurrences happens. At times, the memories may be vivid but there may be lack of clarity as to how they are related and the sequence of time. The apparent inconsistencies in the testimony at times even contradictory are not to be seen as conscious attempts to mislead the courts. The concluding part illustrated the mechanisms of splitting the bad and projecting it on the other. As in "I am good – I care for the child" <> "He is bad and does not care for the child." Or finding unbearable guilt and converting "I feel guilty" into "He/She is accusing me." The participants were facilitated to look at instances in their own life experience wherein they could see it at play. Like shouting "I am not getting angry – you are getting angry" in an increasingly angry tone in an argument as an example of splitting and projection. That these processes including the defences which all of us use to varying degrees against distress, observed by the judge at play in the behaviour and testimony of the witness, should not work towards stigma and condemnation of the trauma survivor or prosecution for perjury.

Child testimony and law

The Protection of Children from Sexual Offences, Act 2012 (POCSO) has been enacted in India, with the aim of protecting children from offences of sexual assault, sexual harassment and pornography and provide for establishment of Special Courts for trial of such offences. The legislation is in compliance with the United Nations Convention of Child Rights, which mandates that nations are to take measures to prevent the inducement or coercion of a child to engage in any unlawful sexual activity; the exploitative use of children in prostitution or other unlawful sexual practices and the exploitative use of children in pornographic performances and materials.

The statute places the best interest and well-being of the child as of paramount importance and with the aim to protect children from sexual assault, harassment and pornography; to protect the privacy and confidentiality of the child and ensure healthy physical, emotional, intellectual and social development of the child. POCSO lays down the obligation on the police to determine the need of care and protection and provide medical attention and ensure medical examination. There is a statutory duty to inform the child and his/her guardian about the availability of support services including counselling and the right to legal aid and representation.

Cut to reality throws up a very difficult picture. A child may be questioned half-a-dozen times by multiple agencies. On paper, the investigating personnel as well as the judge presiding on the special POCSO courts are supposed to be specially attuned and trained in the areas of child psychology. In reality, the questioning of the child is done by the same police personnel investigating other crimes and who have little patience and understanding of the area. Similarly, the Special POCSO Courts are in reality the same overworked Sessions Court Judges trying the offences of theft, rape and murder that like a sleigh of hand get designated as POSCO Courts in compliance with the law.

Shukla (2018) observes "Repeated interviews at different locations can be very traumatic for the child and at times can cause much more harm to the distressed child. In addition interviews by persons not trained in forensic interviewing can contaminate memory and distort the child's account and may be detrimental in arriving at the truth in investigations." The Youth Justice and Criminal Evidence Act, 1999 (YJCEA) in the United Kingdom provides pointers for the way forward in the context of the Indian legal system. Taking on board the stress, anxiety and fear the YJCEA lays down measures to facilitate the process of evidence in the case of vulnerable and intimidated witnesses titling it as *Special Measures and Directions in case of Vulnerable and Intimidated Witnesses* as well as for *Examination of Witnesses through Intermediaries* (Special Measures).

The court determines if a witness is eligible for the Special Measures. Witnesses under 18 years of age, victims of sexual offences and domestic abuse, domestic and work circumstances, social and cultural background and ethnic origins evoking fear and distress are the factors taken into account in the determination of an individual as a vulnerable or intimidated witness. The Special Measures available include screens (section 23 YJCEA); live link (section 24 YJCEA); evidence given in private (section 25 YJCEA); removal of wigs and gowns by judges and barristers (section 26 YJCEA); Video Recorded Interview (section 27 YJCEA); pre-trial recorded cross-examination (section 28 YJCEA); intermediaries (section 29 YJCEA) and aids to communication (section 30 YJCEA).

If, for example, the court feels the measure of screens would enhance the quality of evidence then screens would be placed either around the witness box or around the dock to prevent the witness from having to see the defendant and the defendant from seeing the witness. The witness will still be seen by others in the court including the judge, jury, lawyers, barristers, interpreter, intermediary and, in some courts, the public gallery. In case of the Special Measure of Live Links Witnesses giving evidence via a live video link outside the courtroom (either from within the court centre, from another court centre or from a remote location) generally only see the judge and the lawyer asking questions. On occasion, witnesses may see other people in the courtroom. Unless the court can also screen the defendant, it is likely that the defendant will be able to see the witness on the screens in the court. The setting aside of wigs and gowns by judges and barristers is another measure to make the atmosphere less intimidating for the witness. In the context of leading and aggressive questioning by the barrister of the accused, the intermediary brought into the picture to assist in making the best available evidence to the court can raise their hand if they feel the child may agree to the information though it is incorrect.

In India under the Protection of Children from Sexual Offences Act, 2012 (POCSO) and the rules made thereunder, there are more or less similar provisions. The Achilles heel in India has been the operationalization and working of the provisions. The workshop I had occasion to attend on the "Introduction to Intermediary Work" in the United Kingdom was conducted by a Registered Intermediary, Trainer, Speech and Language therapist, Forensic Interviewer with expertise in autism and Maxime Cole, Qualified Youth Worker and Forensic Interviewer, who works with children and young people.[7] In India under the POCSO Rules, 2020 under Rules 2(f)[8] and 4(9), there is provision of "Support person" to assist the child in the investigation and trial process. The qualifications and skills remain unspecified and it merely says "a person assigned by the Child Welfare Committee." There is, however, a difference between the provisions on paper and their working in the real world. The statute specifies special knowledge and skill for the judges, prosecutors and investigating staff for POCSO cases along with a specialized cadre with training in psychological understanding of trauma and child development in case of minors as witnesses, In real terms it is the same court room, the same judge who tries regular cases who is designated under the POCSO Act and the same regular prosecutors and police. The Manual developed by the National Institute of Mental Health and Neurosciences (NIMHANS) and the Karnataka Judicial Academy (2019) is illustrative of the state of affairs "Unfortunately, the so-called child-friendly courts in some parts of the country are nothing but a replica of the regular adult court i.e. a large room with the judge sitting at a height, and distant from the witness box/stand, a table at the lower where lawyers gather. A colorful sofa in the witness box really does not change the intimidating nature of the court. Such large spaces with the judge sitting at a higher level than the child, and at a considerable distance from the child, only serves to heighten the fear and distress of the child during trial processes" (p. 50).

Collective traumas

There were large-scale killings and violence at the time of the partition of India in 1947 and there have been a number of killings based on community identity: the anti-Sikh riots in 1984; the trail of killings in 1992 after the demolition of Babri Masjid; the anti-Muslim carnage in 2002 in Gujarat; incidents of public lynching, the killings by private armies of landlords and upper castes of the poor and lower-caste people in India. Arora (2015) observes "India has had a long history of horrific mass crimes committed against specific religious and ethnic groups. The history of what can be called mass crimes or crimes against collectivities of people can be traced back to the partition of India when Muslims, Sikhs and Hindus were both the perpetrators and victims of violence on a massive scale." Invariably, the legal system failed to deliver any semblance of justice in instances of singling out and violence against a group.

The Indian Penal Code, 1860 rechristened Bharatiya Nyaya Sanhita, 2023, in an effort to shed the colonial yoke, is geared mainly for offences in the nature of individual crimes. In cases of mass-scale violence against targeted groups based on religion, caste or race or by state agencies in efforts to crush social movements, the legal system is ill equipped and fails to deliver justice. In the arena of the psyche, the impact and dynamics of collective trauma perhaps may be at variance with those of individual trauma. Individual experiences may get mixed up and conflated with stories of others leading to certain cloudiness in the testimony and inconsistencies, which makes the testimonies unreliable in law and may cast doubt on the integrity of the victim-survivor. There was a limited attempt to address the lacunae and the Communal Violence (Prevention, Control and Rehabilitation of Victims) Bill, 2005 was drafted as a measure in case of violence against a group, caste or community. However, the draft statute did not get enacted into law and need not detain us for the purposes of this paper.

Unfortunately in India, psychoanalysis though in existence for more than a hundred years and having borne witness to the traumatic experiences of the partition of the Subcontinent into India and Pakistan remained almost exclusively in the clinic. The Indian Psychoanalytical Society founded in 1925 is headquartered in Kolkata – a centre for large-scale movements for social change towards a more egalitarian society – yet had no interface with these efforts. In a similar vein, psychoanalysis engaged little with the social ills, malaises and violence in Indian society like dowry deaths, "honor" killings and domestic violence.

The impact of trauma on the psyche in times of peace and war lies at the heart of psychoanalysis. Freud lived through the First World War 1914–1918 and deeply engaged with the role that psychotherapy could play, observes (1919) "Apart from this, the war neuroses are only traumatic neuroses, which as we know, occur in peace time too after frightening experiences or severe accidents, without any reference to a conflict in the ego" (p. 209). Dr. Ernest Simmel, a German doctor worked at a hospital in Posen, a former Prussian province in the German Empire, which is at present Poznan in Poland and worked with soldiers with war neurosis wrote a pamphlet (1918) "War Neuroses and Psychic Trauma, Their Mutual Relations, Presented on the Basis of Studies in Psychoanalysis and Hypnosis."[9] Freud (1955[1920]) "As a result of this publication, the next Psycho-Analytical Congress held in Budapest in September, 1918, was attended by delegates of the German, Austrian and Hungarian Army Command, who promised that Centres should be set up for the purely psychological treatment of war neuroses" (p. 210).

Perhaps, the suggestion of the 1918 Budapest International Psychoanalytical Association to set up centres for the treatment of war neuroses is a pointer to a possible direction. In addition to sensitization and minimization of biases of judges, investigative agencies and prosecutors, perhaps a constructive avenue to explore may be the setting up dedicated centres for the psychological therapeutic treatment in case of individual and collective trauma along with interfacing with the legal system for effective justice in incidents of individual and collective violence.

Notes

1 ZahiraHabibullah Sheikh & Anr vs State of Gujarat & Ors on 8 March 2006.
2 Section 12 of the Contempt of Court Act, 1971: Punishment for contempt of court. – (1) Save as otherwise expressly provided in this Act or in any other law, a contempt of court may be punished with simple imprisonment for a term which may extend to six months, or with fine which may extend to two thousand rupees, or with both:
Provided that the accused may be discharged or the punishment awarded may be remitted on apology being made to the satisfaction of the Court
3 A listing of caste violence is outside the scope of the present paper. A few instances are mentioned below: Kilvenmani Massacre, Tamil Nadu (1968): 44 Dalit laborers burnt alive by landlords; Dehuli Massacre, Uttar Pradesh (1981): 24 Dalits killed by Thakurs; Tsundur Massacre, Andhra (1991): 8 Dalits killed by higher caste Reddys; BathaniTola Massacre, Bihar (1996): 21 Dalits killed by the RanvirSena (a militia of upper-caste landlords) and Laxmanpur Bathe Massacre, Bihar (1997): 58 Dalits killed by upper caste militia.
4 See Shukla (2014). The rage of angels: anger, fury, brutal rape, protests, police action.
5 See Shukla (2019) "Quest for justice: psychoanalytical explorations with judges"
6 For the application of the psychoanalytical perspective to the area of minimizing biases, prejudices and stereotypes in the judicial decision making process see: Shukla, R. Quest for justice – psychoanalytical explorations with judges.
7 For a detailed account of the role of intermediaries to facilitate Achievable Best Evidence to the court and aids to communication see: Shukla (2018). Vulnerable witnesses and criminal justice system - the role of intermediaries.cc
8 Rule 2 (f) of the POCSO Rules, 2020: "support person" means a person assigned by the Child Welfare Committee, in accordance with Sub-rule (7) of Rule 4 to render assistance to the child through the process of investigation and trial, or any other person assisting the child in the pre-trial or trial process in respect of an offence committed under the act.
9 https://shs.cairn.info/journal-psychotherapies-2020-4-page-275?lang=en

Bibliography

Arora, Aditya P. 2015. Genocide – An Indian Perspective. https://www.lawctopus.com/academike/genocide-indian-perspective/. Retrieved 13 November 2025.

Brewin, R. 1989. Cognitive change processes in psychotherapy. Psychological Review, Vol. 96, pp. 379–394.

Communal Violence (Prevention, Control and Rehabilitation of Victims) Bill, 2005. chrome-extension://efaidnbmnnnibpcajpcglclefindmkaj/ https://www.mha.gov.in/sites/default/files/CommunalViolence.pdf. Retrieved 13 November 2025.

Criminal Law Amendment Act, 2013. https://www.indiacode.nic.in/bitstream/123456789/15357/1/criminal_law_ammend_act_2013.pdf. Retrieved 23 October 2025.

Freud, S. 1955[1920]. Memorandum on the electric treatment of war neurotics. Revised Standard Edition, XVII.
Justice, Verma, J.S. (2013). Committee on amendments to criminal laws relating to safety and security of women. https://xn–i1b5bzbybhfo5c8b4bxh.xn–11b7cb3a6a.xn–h2brj9c/sites/default/files/2022-08/JS-VermaCommittee-2013%5B1%5D.pdf. Retrieved 23 October 2025.
Law Commission of India 84th Report on "Rape and Allied Offences: Some Questions of Substantive Law, Procedure and Evidence". https://cdnbbsr.s3waas.gov.in/s3ca0daec69b5adc880fb464895726dbdf/uploads/2022/08/2022080544.pdf. Retrieved 23 October 2025.
Mittal, G. (2009). Virender versus State of NCT of Delhi.2009 (4) Journal of Criminal Cases 2721. New Delhi: Arora Book Agency.
Padampriya P. and Alagesen, M. 2024. Silent sufferers: long-term impact on physical and mental health of child sexual abuse survivors. https://conferencias.ageditor.ar/index.php/sctconf/article/view/869. Retrieved 26th January 2026.
Roth, Newman, Pelcovitz, van der Kolk, and Mandel. 1997. Journal of Traumatic Stress, Vol 10, No. 4, 1997. https://www.academia.edu/3136047/Complex_PTSD_in_victims_exposed_to_sexual_and_physical_abuse_Results_from_the_DSM_IV_field_trial_for_posttraumatic_stress_disorder. Retrieved 27th January 2026.
Shukla, R. 2014. The rage of angels: anger, fury, brutal rape, protests, police action. International Journal of Applied Psychoanalytical Studies, Vol. 11, No. 2, pp. 184–187.
Shukla, R. 2015. Trauma survivors meet the law: explorations in India. International Journal of Applied Psychoanalytical Studies, Vol. 13, No. 3, pp. 271–275 (2016).
Shukla, R. (2018). https://www.livelaw.in/vulnerable-witnesses-and-criminal-justice-system-role-of-intermediaries.
Special Measures and Directions in case of Vulnerable and Intimidated Witnesses as well as for *Examination of Witnesses through Intermediaries*. https://www.cps.gov.uk/prosecution-guidance/special-measures. Retrieved 6 November 2025.
Talwar, Shivangi. 2024. Improving psychosocial interventions for adult survivors of childhood sexual abuse in South Asia. https://discovery.ucl.ac.uk/id/eprint/10206027/1/Talwar_10206027_Thesis_Redacted.pdf. Retrieved 26th January 2026.
Youth Justice and Criminal Evidence Act, 1999. https://www.legislation.gov.uk/ukpga/1999/23/contents. Retrieved 6 November 2025.
ZahiraHabibullah Sheikh &Anr vs State of Gujarat & Ors on 8 March, 2006. https://indiankanoon.org/doc/105430/. Retrieved 23rd January 2026.

5 Inner World of Judges

Psychoanalytical Explorations

The promise of law is the deliverance of impartial justice. Law as a discipline stresses rationality, logic and intellect and as a consequence, a considerable body of jurisprudence has developed to check arbitrariness, which is regarded as the anti-thesis of equality in human actions. All of us in an osmosis-like process tend to imbibe to a greater or lesser degree, the biases, prejudices and stereotypes of the race, community, caste, religion, gender and class, in which we have been raised. Legal systems assume that an individual appointed as judge functions impartially, but there is unfortunately no way of being miraculously free from prejudices, biases and stereotypes. Likewise, the apprehensions, anxieties and fears of the individual judge are as likely to impact the working and interpretation of laws. The disjunction between the judiciary and the predominant majority of the persons caught in the legal machinery, especially those from the lower socio-economic classes, the subordinate castes and the subaltern tribes and communities in India, further impacts the inequitable working out of law.

A case in point is the recent nationwide uprising in India by the marginalized and exploited communities, the Scheduled Castes (SCs) and Scheduled Tribes (STs), who have historically been discriminated against in India. The SCs and STs are listed in a specific schedule of the Constitution of India in order to correct centuries of inequality. Vigorous protests by these communities took place in April 2018 against a Supreme Court judgment perceived to be diluting the special law, the Scheduled Castes and Tribes (Prevention of Atrocities) Act, 1987 (SC/ST Act) according to which perpetrators of atrocities against these subaltern sections could not get anticipatory bail from courts. The headlines in national dailies read '9 die as massive Dalit protests across country turn violent'[1] or 'SC's dilution of SC/ST Act caused great damage'[2] and are indicative of the gap between the marginalized populations and the Indian judiciary. *Dalit* – which literally means 'oppressed' in several Indian languages – is an empowering term used by the political movements of the castes at the bottom of the caste hierarchy including former 'untouchables'.[3] A pointer to the relationship of the judiciary to caste is the recent Bombay High Court directive to the Ministry of Information and Broadcasting and the

DOI: 10.4324/9781003626794-6

Press Council of India to issue an advisory to the media to avoid the word '*dalit*' in their reports.[4] There is very little representation in the judiciary of the communities affected by these rulings. The National Commission for Schedule Castes in 'A Report on Reservation in Judiciary' notes "Even today in 2011 there are only 24 judges belonging to SC/STs against a total of 850 judges in all the 21 high courts, but 14 out of the 21 high courts do not have a single SC/ST judge. Similarly, there is not a single judge belonging to SC/STs in the Supreme Court where the strength of judges is 31" (p. 7).

There are sections in any society who proclaim their hatred against particular categories of persons as their agenda. In a polarizing trend, there is increasing loud articulation of hate and lynching of Muslims in some parts of India by Hindu extremist organizations formed with the conscious agenda of hierarchies based on religion, with Hindu supremacy a guiding force. In a similar vein, there are upper-caste organizations with a proclaimed agenda of caste superiority. However, an exception or two apart, few judges would consciously think, 'I am against workers' or 'I think Muslims are bad' or 'homosexuals are disgusting', yet these ingrained notions impact judicial behaviour and functioning. The seeds of biases, prejudices and origins lie in and operate at an unconscious level. However, there is no formal acknowledgement by the legal systems the world over, of the role of the unconscious in law. Yet, in practice, any encounter with the legal system inevitably brings home the bearing of the unconscious and the irrational in law. Seasoned lawyers from experience know the impact of the visual image on the judge. In matrimonial disputes, lawyers routinely advise the woman not to wear her 'Sunday best' for court appearances as the sight of a well-dressed woman may influence the quantum of money fixed by the judge as maintenance from the husband. In turn, the husband may well be advised to present a pitiful appearance before the court to evoke sympathy so as not have to pay a high monthly maintenance to his wife.

Apart from decisions in specific disputes or the determination of guilt or innocence of an individual accused of an offence, the impact of the unconscious can be seen in almost all spheres of law. Human rights jurisprudence, constitutional validity of legislations to the very drafting and working of the laws seem majorly impacted by the unacknowledged irrational and unconscious. Taking Freud's (1905) conception in the context of 'dream work', the psychoanalytic frame offers us pointers to move from the 'manifest' to the 'latent' in law.

The question of shared assumptions

In the arena of psychoanalysis, phrases like 'conscious' and 'unconscious', 'affect' and 'associations' are commonly used, based on shared assumptions and premises. However, the minute we take the frame to another field, the assumptions can no longer be taken to be universal. In a sense, the basic principles or premises of psychoanalysis have to be first established through everyday experiences of persons.

Many of us as lawyers, litigants or observers in court may have witnessed or been a party to an irritable exchange between the judge and a lawyer. All of us are human and irritation, anger, frustration and perceived provocation influence rational thought. At times, the judge may be heard to observe that he/she never lets such exchanges with counsel impact the adjudication on the merits of the case to the detriment of the interests of the parties involved in the litigation. This could be due to the image of a judge as a person unaffected by emotions in the discharge of judicial functions. This self-image may make a thought like: "as a judge I get affected by angry exchanges" intolerable, and the thought gets suppressed and denied at a conscious level. The suppressed emotions impact mental functioning and the discharge of judicial duties. Almost everyone else present in court, barring the judge, senses *"Judge sahib naraz ho gaye hain"* (trans. the judge has become angry) and a price may have to be paid.

A more meaningful paradigm could be to acknowledge the feelings engendered by the angry exchange and take them on board at the conscious level. Feelings which are suppressed are not amenable to processing and yet continue to impact human actions. Once feelings are in the conscious domain, they can be processed in the psyche. A judge after acknowledging feelings of irritability may take a sip of water and think, "Maybe it is better not to pass a final order today" or "Maybe I should adjourn this case today" or "Maybe I should *recuse* myself from this case." It makes possible conscious choice to reduce the impact of the angry-irritable feeling engendered by the exchange, which could adversely affect adjudication on the merits of the case.

Opening Windows

It is these everyday examples that help in opening the window towards the movement from the manifest conscious to the hidden unconscious. A special responsibility rests on individuals placed in judicial positions to try and reduce the impact of personal biases, prejudices and stereotypes in order to promote impartiality. Gender, caste, class, race, religion, nationalism and sexual orientations are some of the likely areas of play of these notions.

Judicial training is oriented towards following and being guided by the observations and judgments of superior courts. Fortunately, in a first, the Supreme Court of India in a judgment has acknowledged the possibility of unconscious prejudice on the part of the judges.[5] The Punjab and Haryana High Court had ordered the termination of the pregnancy of an adult woman who had not given her consent for the procedure. The woman had been categorized as 'mentally retarded', and consent was deemed to be irrelevant. Reversing the High Court order, the Honourable Chief Justice of India (CJI) observed: "...this case also presents an opportunity to confront some social stereotypes and prejudices that operate to the detriment of mentally retarded persons. Without reference to the present proceedings, *we must admit that even medical experts and judges are unconsciously susceptible to these prejudices*" (emphasis the author's). The CJI went on to perceptively observe: "It would also be proper to emphasize that persons who are found to be in a condition of borderline, mild or moderate mental retardation are capable of being good parents."

Psychoanalysis and the Mexican judicial experiment

In talking of psychoanalysis and law, it is fitting to discuss the experiment of Judge Carrancá in Mexico, about whom Gallo (2012) observes, "One of the most original and eccentric readers Freud had anywhere in the world was Raúl Carrancá y Trujillo, a Mexican judge who studied in Spain, returned to Mexico City in the 1930s, and worked tirelessly to reform the judicial system by, in part, incorporating psychoanalytical ideas into the legal profession" (p. 253).

Carranca (1934), a Mexican judge and a great admirer of Freud referring to him as 'that intrepid explorer of the human soul and its dark, subterranean recesses' (p. 125), in an unprecedented move, placed defendants who were referred to him in a chair, sat behind them and invited them to explore their fears, fantasies, anxieties, dreams and anxieties in order to arrive at the truth. In the Mexican legal system – unlike the Indian and the British – the judge has investigative functions. The judge published his experiment in the journal *Criminalia*. Gallo (2012) informs us, "Soon after 'A legal experiment with psychoanalytic techniques' appeared in *Criminalia*, Carrancá mailed a copy to Freud. Freud (1934) responded with a gracious – albeit brief – letter, telling the Mexican judge that he had read his article with great interest and approved of the efforts to find new applications for psychoanalysis, and that "it has always been an ideal desire for the psychoanalyst to win two people for our discipline: teachers of youth and judges" (p. 257).

The role of analyst to the defendant played by Judge Carrancá would be impermissible in India, where the role of the judge is that of an impartial referee between adversaries. The inquisitorial system followed in Mexico gave space to Judge Carrancá to play the analyst-therapist to the accused-defendant.

The case of the accused in the famous Leon Trotsky[6] murder case was allotted to Carrancá. The assassin confessed to the crime claiming disillusionment with Trotsky as the motive and the matter could have ended there. However, Judge Carrancá was keen to explore the motive and the identity of the perpetrator who appeared to be using an alias. This time around, the judge rather than conducting the analysis himself directed a criminologist and a forensic psychiatrist to explore the unconscious motives of the assassin.

Freud died in 1939 and would have turned in his grave at the verdict in the Trotsky case in 1943 holding 'Oedipus Complex' as the motive for the murder. When called upon to give an expert opinion in the Halsmann case, Freud (1931) writes "Precisely because it is always present, the Oedipus Complex is not suited to provide a decision on the question of guilt" (p. 252). The inquisitorial system providing leeway for Carrancá to play analyst apart, the use of psychoanalytical tools like free association, the explorations of dreams and fantasies of the accused-defendant and the violation of the basic tenet of confidentiality inherent in the mixing up the judicial and analytical role is unlikely to serve the interests of justice.

Law in Praxis

> *Tu kehta pothi kee lekhi, main kehta ankhan kee dekhi*
> ("You speak that which is written in books, I speak that which is seen by the eye")
>
> Kabir[7]

Incarceration in jail involves the curtailment of the vital rights to life and liberty of the individual. The essential principles of Anglo-Saxon jurisprudence like 'presumption of innocence', 'burden of proof on prosecution', 'objective evaluation of evidence' and 'proving beyond reasonable doubt' were evolved and crystallized over time and are irreproachable. In practice, these high principles of law are played out in hundreds of courtrooms in India, mediated through the agency of a judge, an individual as much prey to human foibles, idiosyncrasies, pride, prejudices and egotism.

A person arraigned for theft may in appearance fit the very stereotype of a drug addict in the mind of the judge and evoke a gut feeling, *'smackiya hai, isi ne chori kee hogi'* ('the guy is a smack addict, must have committed the theft'). The 'gut feeling' impacts and influences in a vital manner the application of the legal principles like the presumption of evidence, the evaluation of evidence and the determination of innocence or guilt in the theft case. However, judicial training does not have any component of taking this gut feeling 'on board', in the sense of acknowledgement, awareness and processing of the feelings evoked with a view to a fair application of the legal maxims to the case of the apparent 'drug addict' already condemned as guilty, even before the start of the trial and presentation of evidence to establish the offence.

Apart from individual cases, the unconscious at play can be seen in the adjudication of the constitutional validity of laws touching upon nationalism, gender and sexuality including sexual orientation. National security laws in India, such as the 'Terrorist and Disruptive Activities (Prevention) Act', 1985 in the Kartar Singh (1995) case,[8] the 'Prevention of Terrorism Act', 2002[9] and the 'Armed Forces (Special Powers) Act', 1956,[10] which impact civil liberties and democratic rights have been challenged in the courts but have been consistently upheld as constitutionally valid by the Supreme Court of India. The judgments delivered by the courts upholding the laws are on the manifest level about aspects of the fundamental rights to life, liberty, freedom of speech and expression and reasonable restrictions to be imposed on these rights on the ground of public morality, public order and national security. Love for mother and motherland; anxieties of disintegration of the country, particularly poignant in the context of the partition of India in 1947 and the internal imago of the brave son of Mother India in the psyche of the judges are some of the unacknowledged factors that impact the adjudication of constitutionality of such laws.

Yet, judges by definition are deemed to be free from personal biases, prejudices and stereotypes as soon as they occupy the judicial chair. Healy (1950) reviewing Courts on Trial, Myths and Reality in American Justice by Jerome Frank observes "The virile chapter on The Cult of the Robe shows what Judge Frank is after, namely, to have an intelligent public understand 'that the springs of decision in judges' do not 'differ from the springs of decision in other men'. The wearing of the robe and legal jargon tend to becloud that fact" (p. 238). What then are the possibilities of intervention?

Affect and free association workshops

Applying the psychoanalytic frame giving primacy to 'affect' followed by 'free association', I conducted a series of workshops on 'Minimizing the impact of biases, prejudices and stereotypes in the judicial-decision making process', at the National Judicial Academy, Bhopal; the Delhi Judicial Academy, New Delhi and the Karnataka Judicial Academy, Bengaluru in India. The workshops were targeted at newly recruited judges as well as senior judges attending refresher courses. The senior judges had been in service for up to 15–20 years.

We begin with open-ended queries about individuals who feel they are totally free from biases and prejudices to those feeling a little biased and prejudiced. It is rare for a participant to take up the gauntlet of being an extremely prejudiced individual. Participants volunteer to share and mention the biases they are aware of and we proceed to establish the distinction between conscious and unconscious biases.

Predominantly, images and words were projected on the screen and in the first round, the participant-judges were to get in touch with the feelings. The judicial role being cerebral, getting in touch with one's feelings and articulating them require effort on the part of the individual and is one of the objectives of the workshop. In the second round of reactions, the participants were to express the associations to the images. The images selected were keeping in mind the intersection of class, caste, gender, sexuality and sexual orientation. Some of the images projected on the screen were: Mother; Black; White; Peaceful Protest Picture; Criminal; Bearded Keffiyeh Man; Man inhaling from foil; Schedule Caste; Sexy Woman; Homosexual; Dowry; Celebrity, Naxalite[11] and Fair Handsome Man. As illustrative, we take up responses to three of the images projected on the screen.

Mother and bearded Keffiyeh[12] man

The image depicting or symbolizing 'Mother' evoked feelings of 'Care, Affection, Comfort, Respect, Obedience, Security, Devotion, Patience, Pride, Sacrifice, Strength, Pamper, Kindness, Compassion, Happy, Nurturance and Solicitude'. The image of a bearded man with a keffiyeh evoked feelings of 'Suspicion; Fear; Anger; Terror; Curiosity; Hate; Caution; Contempt; Shock; Surprise; Aggression; Worry; Horror and Anxiety'.

The free associations of the participants to 'Mother' were in the nature of: 'Great sense of security; My mother; Life's First teacher; Can endure anything; Most respected; Goddess; Guiding light; Missing her; Food; Guidance; She is one who created; Energy of life; Scolding; '*Dantna*' (trans. scolding); Selfless; Our Mother; Responsible; Dedicated; Teaching me religious things; Most Lovable; Should be respected; Sacrifice; Ask for anything; Life-giving soul; Life-giving teacher'.

The free associations of the participants to the Bearded Keffiyeh Man were 'Muslim; Fundamentalism; Arab; Basketball player; Looks like a terrorist; Needs help; Needs to be put behind bars; Osama; '*Kattar*' (trans. hardcore); Who is he looking at?; Thank God he is not staring at me; Terrorist; *Akshardham*[13]; Criminal; Threatening; Needs to be educated; Orthodox; Human beings; Fanatic; Belief in own religion; 'band' (trans. Closed); Desperate; Son of Osama bin Laden; Directionless; Needs help; Insecurity; Religious man; What is he up to?; *Intifada*; *Al-Qaeda*; Cruel; Religious identity; Dissatisfied; Terror will he create; Harm; Explosives; Creation of God; Allah; Pious; Cleric; Distance; Curious who is he; Ghetto. 'In a somewhat similar vein', the word 'Naxalite', referring to the armed left-wing revolutionary movements in India, evoked feelings of Terror; Fear; Dilemma; Anger; Sympathy; Hatred; Repulsion; Curiosity; Injustice; Pity; Insecurity; Hate; Violence; and Anguish.

At the level of 'affect', the feelings evoked by Mother and Bearded Keffiyeh Man seem to fall into neat categories: All the positive feelings with the Mother image and the negative with the Bearded Keffiyeh Man. The value-loaded sharpness of the contrast was similar to feelings evoked by the two colours Black and White. At the level of free associations, the Scolding Mother is the closest to a negative. In the case of the Bearded Keffiyeh Man, the most benign associations were basketball player, Pious, Creation of God, and at the other end of the spectrum were Hate, Osama, Cruel and Create terror.

The participant-judges were invited to share their experiences of trying accused under anti-terror laws and for offences like sedition. Sharing of feelings by the participants of anxiety and/or fear evoked at setting eyes on an accused individual who fits the very stereotype of a 'terrorist' helped in weaving in the inter-connections between the emotions and the free associations evoked in the workshop and the possible impact of their feelings on the trial process. Participants sharing the mobilization of positive feelings of love, affection, security for life-giving mother and motherland along with the negative feelings of horror, fear and terror evoked by the Bearded Keffiyeh Man assist in illustrating the playing out of these emotions in courtrooms.

Unconscious fears of rape and pillage by gun-toting 'Terrorists' and 'Naxalites' and fantasies of the brave 'Lion' son protecting mother and motherland appear to play their role in the apparent objective processes of legal trials. Baccheta (2004) writes, "As Andrew Parker et al. [1992] have amply demonstrated, in so many nationalisms across the globe the territorial component is associated with, or symbolised as, a chaste female body, often a mother or motherly figure. The notion of her potential violation by foreign invaders is also widespread" p. 27). I elsewhere observe "The vague inimical forces get reified in the stereotype of the bloodthirsty bearded AK-47 toting "terrorist" out to destroy. Childhood fantasies of protecting mother against the bad father may mesh in with those of the macho boy soldier and brave patriot son defending the Mother Nation. The plethora of feelings which may get provoked impact fair, balanced and rational application of mind with regard to the validity of such laws" (Shukla, 2011, p. 349).

'Unnatural Sex' and homosexuality

An image depicting two men holding hands in an apparent homosexual relation evoked the following feelings: Sick; Deprived; Not again; Abnormal; Aversion; Repulsive; Helplessness; No feeling; Neutral; Secrecy; Lust; Bad; Empathy; Ignore; Compassion; Passion; Disgust; Deviance; Discomfort; Sympathy; Hatred; Uncomfortable; Inhuman; Revulsion; Confusion; Pity; Blank; and Curiosity.

Coming to thoughts, the free associations of the participant judges were: Proper treatment; Love and care; Getting between; Delhi High Court; Discouragement; Defiance; Deviation; Perversion; Each his own; HIV; Latest issue; Let them live; Social stigma; Legalize their; Offence against nature; Gender; Transgender; Hostel; Unnatural; Psycho; Abnormal; Diseased; Ailment; Difference; Their own wish; Interference; Accepting variety; Shameful; How could they enjoy it?; Distorted; Aberrations; Deviants; Abnormal; Discrimination; Naz Foundation; Type of sex; Unusual; Justice Murali; Immoral; Unnatural; Illegal; Feeling of person; Justice Shah; Adverse to nature; Mental sickness; and Different people.

The Indian Penal Code, 1860, drafted by the British criminalized homosexuality under Section 377 as 'unnatural sex'. The Delhi High Court in a landmark judgment in the *Naz Foundation case* in 2009 excluded homosexual sex among consenting adults from the ambit of the offence. However, the Supreme Court in appeal overturned the verdict in the *Surendra Kumar Kaushal case* in 2014 and held Section 377 of the IPC to be constitutionally valid and applicable even to consensual adult homosexual acts, again rendering a significant section of society as 'criminals'. After a wait of five long years, the Supreme Court in the recent judgment of 6th September 2018 in the dancer-choreographer *Navetej Singh Johar (2016) case* has reversed its own earlier judgment terming it as 'arbitrary, fallacious and retrograde' and held criminalizing consensual acts between adults as unconstitutional. The flip-flops give us an indication of the powerful role that subjective factors in the psyche of a judge may play in adjudicating on merits in the apparent legal paradigm of fundamental rights to life, liberty, equality, speech and expression and constitutionally permissible reasonable restrictions.

The conscious and unconscious notions of the individuals performing the judicial function about 'natural–unnatural sex'; heterosexuality-homosexuality-bisexuality; 'normal sex'–'abnormal sex' impact adjudication in this arena. Feelings of disgust at homosexuality and penalizing homosexual acts among consenting adults may well stem from unacknowledged homosexual attractions of an individual. Lack of acknowledgement of one's own homosexual inclinations could impact decisions in the arena of sexuality. Reaching a certain minimal comfort level with regard to sexuality, processing anxieties about differences and diversities in the area of gender identity and sexual orientation are a sine qua non for a balanced judicial temperament. These factors also come into play in cases involving the validity of exclusion of marital rape from the offence of rape or the issue of adultery as an offence or the validity of the non-prosecution of the woman under the adultery law, issues presently under challenge in the Supreme Court of India.

Caste and psyche

According to traditional Hindu thought, there are four castes with the *Brahmin* originating from the head, the *Kshatriya* from the arms, the *Vaishya* from the thighs and the *Shudras* from the feet. The hierarchy corresponds to the correlates of Knowledge, Defence, Sustenance and Service, respectively.

Caste, which is a unique and predominant feature of Indian society, transcends the Hindu religion and has permeated Christianity, Islam and Sikhism. It is both blatant and lurking under the surface and is generally accessible to most Indians at all times. It is a volatile and sensitive issue today and in the workshops with judges, caste remained the most difficult area in which to access emotions evoked in the participants. Leaving aside an exception or two, participants chose to give politically correct answers. Judges trying cases under anti-discriminatory laws like the Protection of Civil Rights Act, 1956 and The Scheduled Castes and Scheduled Tribes (Prevention of Atrocities) Act, 1989 are trying with the full force of conscious logic and rationality at their command to be impartial. Yet, the judgments and interpretations of the provisions of the two legislations in the cases reflect the unconscious caste biases.[14]

The complaint of Justice Karnan of the then Madras High Court to the National Commission of Schedule Castes in 2011 came in useful as an illustration in my attempts to access and process unconscious caste biases in workshops with judges. Justice Karnan, who is a Dalit, complained that: "The judge, sitting cross-legged next to me, touched me with his shoes deliberately and then said sorry. Two other judges were watching it smiling," he said. Justice Karnan claimed that he was discriminated against on the basis of caste at several get-togethers such as full court meeting, high tea and dinner.[15]

The brother judge may have touched his shoe intentionally to humiliate or it may have been accidental. Likewise the two judges may have been watching and enjoying Justice Karnan's humiliation or it may be possible that they might have been smiling at a joke entirely unrelated to Justice Karnan. As a measure to diffuse tensions, Justice Karnan was transferred to Calcutta High Court. However, matters escalated, Justice Karnan accused the seven judges of the Supreme Court bench who issued contempt notice to him, of committing contempt and also 'convicted' them of offences under the SC/ST Act. In a step unprecedented in judicial history, the Supreme Court of India found Justice Karnan guilty of contempt of court and sentenced him to six months' imprisonment. The direction by the Supreme Court for a psychiatric examination of Justice Karnan did not help and seems to have been perceived by the judge as a persecutory attack. In contrast to aspects of psychiatry with mental illness as pathology, perhaps, therapy-counselling sessions from a psychoanalytical approach, which looks upon the 'pathological' as part of the spectrum of the 'normal', may have been a more constructive avenue to explore in Justice Karnan's case.

Individual sessions with judicial officer

From a psychoanalytic approach with an implicit assumption of the availability of an endless number of sessions, I was in a dilemma about taking up an assignment with the limit of a maximum of five sessions of therapy with a judicial officer. Taking inspiration from the colourful Ukrainian proverb '*He who doesn't risk, doesn't drink champagne*', the equivalent of the sedate English proverb 'nothing ventured, nothing gained', I accepted the engagement. The setting was the Judicial Academy and the High Court headed by the Chief Justice, the superintending authority for subordinate judicial officers, had directed re-training of the magistrate. The therapy sessions were being paid for by the Academy, not the judicial officer. Much like concerned parents who want to know about the session of the child, the persons-in-charge met me before and after the session. Assuring confidentiality to the client-magistrate would inspire little confidence under the circumstances. Sensitively, the authorities understood and waived the requirement of meeting them pre- and post-session.

I will attempt to flag some of the issues that arose in the sessions. Legal details like provisions of law and reported judgments of courts including citations in combination with a flowery and convoluted manner of talking took up lot of space in the session. A fascination, almost like a craving or greed for the language and wordplay of law, reflected in a phrase like-'I didn't get satiated' referring to the law course. The pre-occupation with detail and wordplay as a defence to stave off lurking distressful feelings could be an avenue to explore.

Much like the elephant in the room which no one is talking about, there was no mention by the Magistrate of the reason he was here in the session. The leave of the officer had been cancelled as a punitive measure and he was instead sent for training by the Chief Justice. In the sessions, the Chief Justice came across as an inspirational mentoring figure whose approval meant much to the youthful magistrate. Along with feeling that his action was justified, was the emotion that 'they know better' with regard to the punitive measure taken by the authorities. Possibly, the anger or rage fleetingly surfaced as resentment against his father-in-law and against old lawyers appearing before the young magistrate.

As part of judicial training, the motto not to be a 9 am to 5 pm judge, but to be a 24-hour judge was inculcated. This in turn seems to have fed a grandiose self which looked upon colleagues as well as at personnel from investigation agencies with contempt, leading to friction at work. There were also problems in the marriage, though the wife's complaints had been put on hold by the protective Chief Justice. The crisis in the marriage was related in a calm manner without pain and anguish. Possibly, day in and day out using the formal legal language of courts can have a distancing from emotions effect on the personality. Phrases like 'matrimonial relations' instead of 'my marriage' or 'spouse' compared to the intimacy of 'partner' or 'wife' creep and spread into the personal arena. The emotional distancing could play a role and contribute to relationship problems. Given the setting of five sessions as part of a punitive order along with anxiety about the therapist 'spilling the beans', creating a safe, secure, holding space for painful and distressing emotions to play out and work through integral to therapy was difficult to achieve in the circumstances.

Balint groups and individual sessions

Intra-psychic processes like our inner feelings of hostility getting split and converted into perceptions of the 'other' as hostile to us; or denial of our feelings of humiliation leading to perceiving the actions of the other as slights; or suppressed feelings of guilt leading to feelings of being accused are at play in all of us. Judges are the same as the rest of us and there is no reason to suppose that processes of denial, splitting and projection are not at play in them. Freud (1906) cautions that judges may "'be led astray by a neurotic who, although he is innocent, reacts as if he were guilty, because a lurking sense of guilt that already exists in him seizes upon the accusation made in the particular instance' (p. 113). Providing a facilitating space for observing these processes through *Balint groups* equips the individual to better perform the judicial function.

Balint groups initiated by Hungarian-British psychoanalyst Michael Balint were spaces where about eight to ten doctors met at regulator intervals along with a facilitator and one or two cases were presented focusing on the non-medical aspects. *Balint* groups for judges would provide a space not to discuss legal aspects but to explore feelings in a non-judgmental space. It would offer an opportunity to reflect on work as well as a space to articulate anxieties and frustrations. It could lead to increased self-awareness, more capacity to reflect on themselves and the usefulness of examining one's own reactions. To illustrate, a mother who is a judge in child custody matters may find her maternal feelings evoked and invariably feel inclined to give custody to the mother, regardless of the merits. The legal system offers no space for the articulation of the 'non-legal' responses evoked in judges who are as human as anyone else. A space for naming the feeling, elaborating and processing the emotion could lead to improved judicial functioning as well as judges being better equipped to address the psychological aspects of issues like trauma testimony.[16] Experiencing the creativity of a group and greater professional satisfaction could be other possible positive outcomes.

When parents are stressed in their quasi-judicial functions of arbitrating quarrels among children, the quantum multiplier in the stress and strain in deciding life and death matters, day in and day out, cannot be imagined. Healy (1950) observes that Frank (1949) advocates that judges "... should undergo at least a short period of psychoanalysis that they may acquire knowledge of themselves and thereby learn to control to some extent their own otherwise unavoidable preconceptions and biases" (p. 238). Individual therapy sessions for judges would offer spaces to observe biases and prejudices, get in touch with feelings in the nature of slights, humiliation and helplessness as well as take on board feelings of grandiosity and omnipotence. These emotions could thus possibly be processed better and lessen the impact on judicial behaviour and action.

Notes

1 Times of India, 3 April, 2018.
2 Times of India, 13 April 13, 2018.
3 Untouchability was prohibited post-Independence by Article 17 of the Constitution of India, as well as a specific legislation titled 'The Untouchability (Offences) Act' passed in 1955 (renamed in 1976 as 'Protection of Civil Rights Act'). However, untouchability continues to be practiced in several pockets across the country.
4 HC to Govt: Ask media to avoid 'Dalit' word. Times of India, 7 June 2018.
5 Suchita Srivastava versus Chandigarh Administration, 2009 (11) SCALE 813.
6 Trotsky exiled in Mexico was widely suspected to have been assassinated on the directives of Stalin.
7 15th Century mystic poet with biting criticism of Hindu and Islamic practices in couplets referred to as '*dohas*'.
8 Kartar Singh versus State of Punjab (1994) 3 SCC 569.
9 Peoples' Union for Civil Liberties versus Union of India, 2004 (9) SCC 580.
10 Naga People's Movement for Human Rights versus Union of India (1998) 2 SCC 109.

11 The term 'Naxalite' is derived from Naxalbari village in West Bengal, India, the site of an armed peasant revolt in 1967.
12 Traditional headdress in West Asia, originating from Kufa, Iraq typically worn to protect against sunburn, dust and sand.
13 Akshardham temple in Gandhinagar, Gujarat, India was attacked by two armed men on 24 September 2002 killing 30 persons.
14 For examples of caste bias reflected in judgments under the two anti-discriminatory laws see 'Judicial Pronouncements and Caste' by Shukla (2006).
15 Dalit judges targeted, says Justice Karnan. Times of India, 4 November 2007.
16 For trauma testimony and law, see 'Trauma survivors meet the Law: Explorations in India'. Shukla (2016).

Bibliography

Baccheta, P. 2004. Gender in the Hindu Nation, RSS women as ideologues. New Delhi. Women Unlimited (an associate of Kalifor Women).

Carrancá y Trujillo, R. 1934. Un ensayo judicial de la psicotécnica. *Criminalia* Vol. 6, No. Feb, p. 125.

Frank, J. 1949. Courts on Trial. Myths and Realities in American Justice. New Jersey: Princeton University Press.

Gallo, Reuben. 2012. A Wild Freudian in Mexico: Raúl Carrancá Y Trujillo. Psychoanalysis and History, Vol. 14, No. 2, pp. 253–267.

Freud, S. 1905. Jokes and their relation to the unconscious. Standard Edition VIII.

Freud, S. 1931. 1930. The Expert Opinion in the Halsmann Case. Standard Edition XXI.

Freud, S. 1934. Letter to Carrancá y Trujillo, 13 February 1934. *Criminalia* 8 (April 1934): 160. (Reproduced in with English translation by Gallo, R (ibid).

Healy, W. 1950. Courts on Trial. Myths and Realities in American Justice by Jerome Frank. Review. Psychoanalytic Quarterly, Vol. 19, pp. 437–438.

Kartar Singh versus State of Punjab. 1994. 3 Supreme Court Cases 569. Eastern Book Company, Lucknow, India.

Naga People's Movement for Human Rights versus Union of India. 1998. 2 Supreme Court Cases 109. Eastern Book Company, Lucknow, India.

A Report on Reservation in Judiciary. National Commission of Schedule Castes. https://ncsc.nic.in/storage/special_events/owpsaxblMRcpFAU0XZaRNTaFxkyG1DI3jEEYt3gX.pdf. Retrieved 09th June 2018.

Naz Foundation v. Govt. of NCT of Delhi. 160 Delhi Law times 277. D.L.T. Publications Private Limited, Delhi, India.

Navtej Singh Johar versus Union of India Writ Petition (Criminal) No. 76 of 2016. https://www.livelaw.in/breaking-sc-strikes-down-157-year-old-law-criminalizing-consensual-homo-sexual-acts-between-adults-holds-section-377-ipc-unconstitutional/. Retrieved 07th September 2018.

Parker, A. et al. (eds). 1992. Nationalisms and sexualities. New York. Routledge.

Peoples' Union for Civil Liberties versus Union of India, 2004 (9) Supreme Court Cases 580. Eastern Book Company, Lucknow, India.

Shukla, R. 2006. Judicial Pronouncements and Caste. Economic and Political Weekly October 21, 2006.

Shukla, R. 2011. Judging Sedition: The Case of the Good Doctor. International Journal of Applied Psychoanalytic Studies, Vol. 8, No. 4, pp. 346–352 (2011).

Shukla, R. 2016. Trauma survivors meet the law: Explorations in India. International Journal of Applied Psychoanalytic Studies, Vol. 13, No. 3, pp. 271–275.

Suresh Kumar Koushal vs. Naz Foundation. 2014. 1 Supreme Court Cases 1. Eastern Book Company, Lucknow, India.

6 "Us" and "Them"

The Psychology of Inter-community Relations

Prologue

The first clashes between the Meitei and Kuki communities broke out on 3 May 2023. The state has been a bubbling cauldron of hatred, violence and killings claiming about 200 lives leading to the fleeing of thousands from their homes. According to data presented by the Inspector General of Police (Operation) I K Muivah earlier this month, over 5,000 cases of arson have been reported, which included more than 4,700 houses that were torched and 386 religious structures that have been vandalized.[1]

Introduction

The present exploration seeks to bring to bear the psychoanalytical gaze to the intra- and inter-psychic processes at play in the context of communal-ethnic-caste conflicts in an effort towards having a loving "us" without needing to have a hated "them." It is an attempt "to replace what is injurious" as Freud puts it and contribute to moving towards better and more harmonious inter-community relations.

Antagonisms, feelings of hostility and resentment between communities are part of everyday existence in the world. Under ordinary times, they may take the shape of cracking pejorative jokes at the other community members while having tea together at the local teashop. There are relationships and friendships among individuals across communities. Similarly, feelings of humiliation and being weak are part of an individuals' existence but remain confined to the verbal sphere and may surface in discussions in the shape of complaints, grievances and verbal swipes at the others. Similarly, there are collective traumas with regard to historical events where there has been no healthy mourning and processing of the perceived hurts and humiliations. In this scenario, the arrival of a charismatic leader, who promises to transform the group and whose strengths and qualities mesh with the emotional needs of the group, impacts the turn of events.

A charismatic leader, who shores up the group identity and esteem by hurting and destroying another group, stokes feeling of humiliations, feeds

DOI: 10.4324/9781003626794-7

into insecurities and anxieties and escalates tensions among the groups. As the communal temperature rises, a person loses or seizes to have an individual identity and is seen totally as a member of the 'enemy' group. Thus, 'A' is seen as a 'Muslim'; 'B' is seen as a 'Hindu'; 'C' is seen as a 'Sikh'; and 'D' is seen as a 'Christian'. The charismatic leader escalates tensions to a boiling point of volcanic eruption. The 'other-enemy' community becomes the repository of all that is bad and demonized and referred to and reduced to "vermin" or "cockroaches" or non-human "beast-like creatures." Killing such creatures does not induce guilt like the killing of a human being. The chapter explores possibilities of healthy mourning and processing of trauma associated with historical events to move towards diminishing the possibilities of malignant use.

The Holocaust during World War II is an illustration of perhaps one of the most extreme examples of the *'othering'* of a community and a determined bid towards its extermination. The ideology, best exemplified by Nazism, postulated the white Nordic Aryan as a 'master' race with Jews and blacks as inferior. The ideology was implemented in Germany by the National Socialist German Workers' Party (the National Sozialistische Deutsche Arbeiterpartei, commonly referred to as the Nazi Party) found its fullest expression under the leadership of Adolf Hitler who led the party from 1933 until his death in 1945. Jews in Germany were systematically deprived of their property and livelihoods as the Nazis brought in laws between 1933 and 1939 to marginalize and disenfranchise Jewish citizens and proceeded to exclude them from professions and commercial life. A decree was passed prohibiting Jews from using public transportation. Jews over the age of six were made by law to mark themselves by wearing the yellow Jewish Star on their outermost garment. Regulations forced Jews to live in designated areas of German cities.[2] The culmination of the "othering" process was the deportation to concentration camps and labour camps, and death in gas chambers.

What could be the underlying factors that prompted and enabled this horrific process? The less unsettling option is the belief that it was some unfortunate predisposition in the German character that made Nazism and the Holocaust possible. In addition to the propaganda of the victors of the war and liberators of those held in concentration camps, a large number of films, novels and comics conveyed the idea that the Germans were 'evil'. Koonz (1987) offers us pointers: "Still, underneath the unique and dated style of Nazism lurked a more universal appeal – the longing to return to simpler times, to restore lost values, to join a moral crusade. What needs drove those millions of "good Germans" willingly into dictatorship, war and genocide?" (p. 18).

Today, with the global rise of cultural nationalism in several countries, the view that the processes that led to the Holocaust were specific to German society in the 1930s is less comforting or even plausible. Freud (1930[1929]) speaking of aggression in humans seems prescient in the context of the decrees seizing the property of Jews and the concentration camps that were to follow, observes: "As a result, their neighbour is for them not only a potential helper or sexual object, but also someone who tempts them to *satisfy their aggressiveness on him, to exploit his capacity for work without compensation, to use him sexually without his consent, to seize his possessions, to humiliate him, to cause him pain, to torture and to kill him*" (emphasis added) (p. 111).

Arendt (1951), German-American political theorist who has examined totalitarianism and authoritarianism, articulates the need for engagement with drives to violence and power and observes, "Yet to turn our backs on the destructive forces of the century is of little avail" (Preface).

Psychoanalysis and social phenomena

The contribution of psychoanalysis to an understanding of the individual psyche is vital and invaluable. The present attempt is in the nature of going to Freud (1921) 'Group Psychology and the Analysis of the Ego' and 'Civilization and its discontents', taking it forward and bringing to bear psychoanalytical approach to social issues. Freud (1930[1929]) in the context of the 'us' and 'them' perceptively observes "It is always possible to bind together a considerable number of people in love, so long as there are other people left over to receive the manifestations of their aggressiveness" (p. 114).

Klaus von Dohnanyi (1986), the Mayor of Hamburg, at the opening ceremony of the 134thInternational Psychoanalytical Association in 1985 at Hamburg pointed out that the International Psychoanalytical Congress held in Wiesbaden in 1932 – "hardly appears to have been aware of the imminent threat posed by National Socialism which, only a few months later, set up in Germany the most brutal dictatorship in human memory" and brought about untold misery and suffering in the world. Mitscherlich (1971), the German psychoanalyst, urged an expansion of horizons and participation in research on collective behaviour of groups otherwise psychoanalysts "will have manoeuvred [themselves] into an isolation of [their] own making" (p. 164).

My own perspectives on these issues have evolved through almost four decades of engagement with movements for social change, which though attempting to move towards a better society, showed a marked reluctance to take on board psychological dimensions of social problems. Jacques (1955) offers clues as to the arduous road to social change when he writes: "From the point of view here elaborated changes in social relationships and procedures call for a restructuring of relationships at the fantasy level, with a consequent demand upon individuals to accept and tolerate changes in their existing patterns of defences against psychotic anxiety. Effective social change is likely to require analysis of the common anxieties and unconscious collusions underlying the social defences determining phantasy social relationships" (p. 498).

Understanding 'Othering'

This chapter seeks to explore and thereby extend possibilities of psychoanalytical insights with regard to intra- and inter-psychic processes being able to constructively contribute towards understanding the phenomenon of 'othering' and moving towards better inter-community relations in India. I use 'community' in the sense that Volkan (2013), who as a psychoanalyst has worked for peaceful co-existence of diverse communities in major conflict areas of the world, uses the term 'large group' referring to persons who share a feeling of sameness and may number in thousands and millions. The identity may be based on markers in the nature of religion, caste, ethnicity, class, language and geographical region among others. Volkan (2013) illustrates the notion by articulations such as: "we are Apaches; we are Lithuanian Jews, we are Kurdish; we are Slav; we are Sunni Muslims; we are Taliban brothers; we are communists" (p. 210). In India, the identity could be religious, whether Hindu, Christian or Muslim; caste, whether Dalit, Other Backward Castes (OBC) or Brahmin; Adivasi, whether Gond or Thangkul. These identities represent a pulling together of diverse threads including shared myths, realities and histories among a host of cultural and political factors.

In phenomena like war, xenophobia, fascism, communalism and genocide – social, economic, political, cultural and psychological factors play a significant role. Akin to the angles of a prism which reveal behind the 'manifest' apparent white light the 'hidden colours', the psychoanalytical perspective is not offered as the single factor explanation, but one of many views of looking at social phenomena. Jost et al. (2003) based on their research in 12 countries in the context of political conservatism posit that given the complexity of human belief systems, a complete explanation is unlikely and that: "The most that can be expected of a general psychological analysis is for it to partially explain the core of political conservatism because the peripheral aspects are by definition highly protean and driven by historically changing, local contexts" (p. 369).

Family constellation

The inculcation of a deep reverence for the mother and father is through a number of folk and mythological stories. According to a popular myth, a competition was announced that whichever god circled the universe fastest would be worshipped first. Ganesha, whose *vahan* (carrier) is a mouse had no chance of winning, given gods who had creatures like tigers and eagles as carriers. Ganesha promptly circled his parents, mother Parvati and father Shiva, representing the whole universe and won the race.

Manifestly, there is utter denial of any ambivalence in the mother-son dyad routinely reflected in Hindi cinema. One of the most famous dialogues of Hindi cinema in a sibling exchange as to respective achievements in life is "*mere paas maa hai*" (trans. I have mother). However, the films of even progressive male directors reflect the denial of ambivalence. A film screened at the film festival on 'Gender and Sexuality' (International Festival on Gender and Sexuality – Identities and Spaces: 12–15 May 2007) in Delhi titled "All about Our Mothers" (Directed by Manak Matiyani and Kuber Sharma, India) is illustrative. The documentary is a portrait of the mothers of the two young male directors. The film brings up issues of housework, role expectations from women, the double burden of working outside and inside the house, but the context/paradigm of the film is exclusively husband-wife relations. It is standard practice in India for a mother to wash the clothes including the undergarments of the sons till marriage when the chore is taken over by the wife. It is implicit that the son old enough to make films will get cooked food on the table and washed underpants. The film has a romanticized portrayal of the "mother-son" relation without a hint of ambivalence, conflict or resentment. The sons are paying a tribute to their mothers and making them "heroines" and the mothers are helping the sons in making the film that eulogizes their role as mothers.

Films and popular media aside, the stories on which a child grows up emphasize the utter selflessness of the mother and total concern for the son with an underlying subtext of potential betrayal or doubt regarding the loyalty of the son, after marriage. "Joru ka gulam" (trans. "Slave-of-the-wife") is one of the commonest sayings to sons who have got married. The implication in the saying is neglect of the mother after marriage.

Splitting, projection, integration

According to traditional Freudian psychoanalysis with regard to stages of development, the child initially does not have the notion of a separate existence from the mother in the first few months of existence. The baby perceives experiences as pleasant or unpleasant, but does not realize that it is the same entity that is experiencing both the satisfying and the frustrating experiences.

The baby is not aware that the fed-admired-secure baby is the same individual as the hungry-rejected-scared baby. At about the age of 36 months, the integration is estimated to take place in the baby that it is the same individual who experiences pleasure and frustration. The baby develops a realistic picture of himself or herself – that he is not entirely 'good' and kind nor entirely 'bad' and cruel. This in turn helps the baby in perceiving other people as integrated individuals too. The baby also develops a more realistic picture of the mother – that the loving mother and the frustrating mother is the same person. The unintegrated bad parts are dealt with unconsciously through repression or externalization that is deposited in things or animals or people outside oneself.

According to Kernberg, Otto in 'Borderline Conditions and Pathological Narcissism, the normal self is a comprehensive whole and represents an integration of contradictory "all good" and "all bad" libidinally invested early self-images. This normal self relates to integrated object representations that have incorporated the "good" and "bad" primitive object representations. Kernberg observes "Therefore, although normal narcissism reflects the libidinal investment of the self, the self actually constitutes a structure that integrates libidinally invested and aggressively invested components; in simple terms, integration of good and bad self-images into a realistic self-concept that incorporates rather than dissociates the various component self-representations is a requisite for the libidinal investment of a normal self. This also explains the paradox that integration of love and hatred is a prerequisite for the capacity for normal love" (p. 316).

Kernberg speaking of normal and pathological narcissism posits that the lack of integrated self generally co-exists with lack of integration of object representations, which are caricatures of "all good" and "all bad." This results in diminished capacity for empathy or for realistic judgment of others, in depth and "behaviour is regulated by immediate perceptions rather than by an ongoing, consistent, internalized model of others, which ordinarily would be available to the self" (p. 317).

In the context of ethno-religious-caste-community tensions, there seems to be universality of the "enemy" other being invariably "dirty" for the dominant community. In rising Nazi Germany – Jews were categorized as 'dirty'; in the context of Hindu-Muslim tensions – Muslims are seen as 'dirty' by Hindus and in the colonial paradigm, the colonial masters designated the natives as 'dirty'. This lack of integration is not confined to feelings of 'dirtiness' alone, but extends to other 'bad' qualities like lust.

The across-the-board prevalence of these dynamics in the context of inter-community tensions and violence raises doubts as to the smooth integration of the "good" and the "bad" in the self-posited in traditional psychoanalytical theory. Perhaps, it is a continuing process at variance with the conception of the integrated 'normal' self by the age of about three years. Volkan (1986) refers to the integrating as 'mending' and observes "*It is my belief (1985a, b) that this integration—which I like to call mending—as well as the repression of the "unmended" units, is never completed,* so it is possible for object relations conflict to continue" (p. 184).

We see a persistent and continuing resistance to acknowledging the 'bad', the 'dirty', the 'lustful' at an individual as well as the collective community level. Perhaps, the sense of being 'good' or possibly 'good enough' is fragile and gets destabilized and threatened by an acknowledgement of the 'bad' in the self. The 'bad' is therefore externalized to outside objects, gets condensed with projection later and may contain devalued aspects of parents. Volkan (1986) posits that "Such "bad" suitable targets contain the precursors of *the concept of an enemy* shared by the group" (p. 185). In a parallel process, some objects, animals or people become the reservoirs of the 'good' aspects of the self – the idealized parts of the parents. For example, to a growing boy in a Hindu household, the cow may become a reservoir of the nurturing, milk feeding and protective mother. In Finland, it may be a sauna that may represent the soothing – idealized mother for the child. Often familiar foods and cultural practices become suitable targets for the externalization of the good aspects. In times of perceived 'threat' or sense of humiliation, these get amplified and, in a sense, louder.

Enemy as reservoirs and narcissism of minor differences

In osmosis like process, the growing child imbibes stereotypes, biases and prejudices prevalent in the community. The mothering or care-taking person helps select durable targets for externalization who become the shared reservoir of the 'bad' parts. Thus for a Muslim child, a 'pig' (the consumption of which is considered *'haraam'* or prohibited in Islam) may be a repository of all 'dirtiness'. A Hindu child growing amidst escalating communal tensions may have the 'Muslim' as the repository of all 'dirt'. The target and reservoir of the unwanted is often 'dirty' and 'smelly' taking on the characteristics of faeces as the child is taught that excreta are dirty. The objects are shared reservoirs for the community. The thought that the other may be like us is intolerable and unacceptable and minor differences acquire a magnitude totally disproportionate to the at times, trivial differences between the two communities.

Freud used the term phrase narcissism of minor differences first in "The Taboo of Virginity" (1918): "... each individual is separated from others by a "taboo of personal isolation," and ... it is precisely the minor differences in people who are otherwise alike that form the basis of feelings of strangeness and hostility between them. It would be tempting to pursue this idea and to derive from this "narcissism of minor differences" the hostility which in every human relation we see fighting successfully against feelings of fellowship and overpowering the commandment that "all men should love one another" (p. 199).

Freud (1930) writing of minor differences observes: "It is clearly not easy for men to give up the satisfaction of this inclination to aggression. They do not feel comfortable without it... it is precisely communities with adjoining territories and related to each other in other ways as well, who are engaged in constant feuds and in ridiculing each other — like the Spaniards and the Portuguese, for instance, the North Germans and South Germans, the English and Scotch, and so on. I gave this phenomenon the name of 'the narcissism of minor differences', a name which does not do much to explain it. We can now see that it is a convenient and relatively harmless satisfaction of the inclination to aggression, by means of which cohesion between the members of the community is made easier" (p. 114).

Relatively harmless to killer rage

The role of the narcissism of minor differences, which at the time was thought of as "relatively harmless satisfaction of the inclination to aggression" by Freud, possibly needs to be explored further in the context of ethnic-religious – national tensions and strife. Many times, an outsider cannot easily distinguish the two conflicting communities whether it may be Gujarati Muslims and Gujarati Hindus or Hutus and Tutsis. Volkan (1986) observes: "In the villages, where usual masculine dress consists of baggy trousers and shirts, the Greeks wear black sashes, the Turks red. In 'normal times' a breach of this colour code might be tolerated, but when ethnic relations are strained, when group cohesion (and therefore individual integrity) is threatened, a Turk would rather die than wear a black sash, and a Greek would be just as adamant in his refusal to wear a red one"(p. 181).

In times of tensions based on any of the indicia in the nature of race, caste, religion – the Community A feels it does not have any similarities with the 'other' Community B and focuses upon and magnifies the minor differences that are bound to exist. Kakar (1995) in his work 'Colours of Violence' illustrates the process of emphasizing the minor differences, imbuing them with heavy emotional content to widen the schism and chasm out and quotes a speech of self-styled Hindu monk Sadhvi Rithambara: "The Hindu writes from the left to right, the Muslim from right to left. The Hindu prays to the rising sun, the Muslim faces the setting sun while praying. If the Hindu eats with the right hand, the Muslim eats with the left. If the Hindu calls India 'mother', she becomes a witch for the Muslim. The Hindu worships the cow, the Muslim attains paradise by eating beef. The Hindu wears a moustache; the Muslim always shaves the upper lip" (p. 165).

Volkan (1986) observes: "So we focus on minor differences, or we create them, in order to strengthen the psychological gap between the enemy and ourselves. The strengthening of the psychological gap is unconsciously obligatory since it serves as a buffer to keep a group's unwanted parts, impulses, and thoughts—which originally belonged to it— from coming back into the group's self" (p. 187).

Inter-se co-operation between members plays a role in the evolution of successful species. This may be particularly true in the case of human beings who lack horns or claws or other features of attack and defence. Erikson speculated that the human species started using the skins, feathers or claws of other animals to protect the defenceless naked body. That on the basis of the specific devices chosen, each tribe, clan or group developed a sense of shared identity and a belief that it alone constituted the human species. Erikson (1966) observed that "Man has evolved (by whatever kind of evolution and for whatever adaptive reasons) in pseudo species, i.e., tribes, clans, classes, etc., which behave as if they were separate species, created at the beginning of time by supernatural intent" (p. 606). In an effort to understand killings among the human species, Volkan (2009) taking Erikson's ideas forward speculates that possibly if large groups felt they belonged to different species, they would kill each other.

Historical and inter-generational trauma

> *We never wanted to burden them with our memories. Jo humhara dukhtha woh hamare tak hi rehta, we wanted the sadness to end with us, to remain in our generation, to never be passed down.*
>
> Malhotra (2022, p. 21)

Historical trauma refers to distressful experiences or events, which occurred in the past impacting a group or community. Unlike trauma that impacts an individual, the traumatic events are suffered by a collective. The infliction of trauma on the group may be based on factors like the religion, ethnicity, caste, sexual orientation or nationality of the collective. Inter-generation trauma refers to trauma that gets passed down from those who lived through the experiences to the succeeding generations.

The Holocaust, the partition of India, the trauma of the forcible taking away of children of indigenous peoples of Canada into government residential schools[3] or the trauma of the caste system which Dalits have endured in India are examples of historical trauma and inter-generational trauma. Children of Holocaust survivors were the first group, in which the impact of the trauma on subsequent generations was studied. Rosenkranz (2015), Holocaust Program – Group Facilitator (2015), observes "In spite of the fact that many survivors chose to remain silent about their experiences, the trauma was ever present"; "It loomed in the air we breathed, like second hand smoke," stated a 62-year-old physician and son of survivors (p. 3). In a similar vein, Malhotra (2022) quotes Indian-Canadian author-actor Lisa Ray whose grandfather and father came to West Bengal at the time of partition in 1947 "What I feel about Partition, even though I haven't lived through it, is real. It's very, very real" (p. xxix).

In the context of the inter-generational trauma of caste, Yengde (2019) speaking of the film India Untouched by K. Stalin (2007) documenting Dalit girl students being forced to clean the premises and bathroom of the school writes: "As I am walking, the mind is stunted and I am constantly thinking about the repeated assaults on Dalit minds that force them to inferiorize their being" (p. 42). In the context of the revolutionary poet Pash line – "*sabse khatarnak hota hai hamare sapno ka mar jana*" (trans. The most dangerous is the death of our dreams), Yengde observes that along with the humiliations and deprivations suffered, the capacity and nature of dreaming gets impacted by the caste system – "Dalit middle-class dreams are yet to mature; for now they exist in the mimicry of the oppressor Other."

Invocation of past trauma

The slogan *"garv se kaho hum hindu hain"* (trans. "Say with pride we are Hindu") struck a chord among a significant number of Hindus, gained much traction and played an important role in mobilizing, perhaps pointing to a continuing sense of humiliation and shame from historical events that occurred hundreds of years earlier. Malhotra (2022) based on a number of interviews across generations of partition survivors observes "that the intensity with which descendants described inherited stories seemed as visceral" and writes "Their second hand connections to these lived traumas and histories went well beyond surface telling into something which has become intrinsically theirs" (p. xxii).

A leader can strike the right chords that awaken and resonate with buried feelings of guilt and emasculation from an event from the past, charismatically bind individuals and catalyse a group to a call for action and revenge for the humiliation of their forefathers through attacking and destroying the "other" group seamlessly conflated with the old attackers of the past. The Somnath temple in the state of Gujarat, India was looted and destroyed in 1025 A.D. by Mahmud of Ghazni. The mythic hero of the epic Ramayana Lord Rama was supposed to have been born in Ayodhya in the state of Uttar Pradesh. It is a common belief that a temple was built on the spot where was Ram was born, which was destroyed and a mosque built by the Mughal emperor Babar in 1528–1529 referred to as Babri Masjid. In 1992 invoking the dual trauma, Lal Krishna Advani, the then Leader of Opposition in the Indian Parliament, started the *Ram Janmabhoomi Yatra* (Journey to reclaim the birthplace of Lord Rama) from Somnath and culminating in the destruction of the Babri Masjid. The Indian Muslims of today became the attacking Mongol hordes of the medieval times as well as the progeny of Babar responsible for destruction of the Ram temple. The invocation by Mr. Advani of the traumatic events evoked strong emotions with an intensity, as if the looting of Somnath and the alleged destruction of the Rama temple had happened a day before and the participants in and along the *Yatra* route were present and saw these long past events themselves, to use an evocative colloquial phrase *"khud apni ankhon se dekha"* (trans. 'saw with my own eyes').

Volkan (1997) describes the invocation by Slobodan Milosevic of the Serbian defeat in Battle of Kosovo in June 1389 by the Ottoman Empire to stoke ethnic tensions and uses the term 'time-collapse' "where people may intellectually separate the past event from the present one, but emotionally the two events are merged." The Bosnian Muslims of today became the Ottoman Turks – the 'enemy' in the chosen trauma of Bosnian Serbs, akin to the conflation of the Indian Muslims with the attacking Mongol hordes in 1025 and the destroyers of the Ram Mandir (Temple) in 1528–1529.

Mourning and memory

> Mourning is regularly the reaction to the loss of a loved person, or to the loss of some abstraction which has taken the place of one, such as one's country, liberty, an ideal, and so on.
>
> *Freud* (1917)

Mourning is a process of grieving for loss and coming to terms with the death of someone precious to us. Events like the partition of India into two countries in 1947 or the abrogation in 2019 of Article 370 of the Constitution of India, which granted special status to the State of Jammu & Kashmir can also evoke feelings of loss in an individual. Mourning helps in coming to terms with the pain and trauma of loss and in that sense can be looked upon as "healthy mourning" rather than pathology. In contrast, melancholia was recognized as a distinct disorder termed "melancholic depression" and is now looked upon as a species of the broad category of major depressive disorders. It is qualitatively different from the term depression as used in ordinary parlance and is characterized by chronic feelings of sadness, lack of interest in anything and may impact performing daily activities like getting out of bed and brushing one's teeth.

Lack of healthy mourning may take us towards melancholia. Freud (1917) enumerating the characteristics of melancholia and mourning as "profoundly painful dejection, cessation of interest in the outside world, loss of the capacity to love, inhibition of all activity, and a lowering of the self-regarding feelings to a degree that finds utterance in self-reproaches and self-reviling, and culminates in a delusional expectation of punishment" and postulates that "The disturbance of self-regard is absent in mourning; but otherwise the features are the same" (pp. 243–244).

Possibly, lack of healthy mourning in the context of historical traumatic may induce feelings of smallness, guilt and shame at a collective level in a community. There were a number of invasions of India in the medieval period. Mahmud of Ghazni invaded India a number of times from 1010 AD onwards and destroyed and looted the Somnath Temple in Western India. Perhaps, not being able to protect Mother India – Bharat Mata – from the lootings, destructions and killings by attackers from medieval times over the years engendered a sense of shame in the Hindu psyche. Bacchetta (2004) writes "As Andrew Parker et al. [1992] have amply demonstrated, in so many nationalisms across the globe the territorial component is associated with, or symbolised as, a chaste female body, often a mother or motherly figure. The notion of her potential violation by foreign invaders is also widespread" (p. 27).

These feelings may at times be evoked by a leader to bind together a community and seek revenge attacking another group conflated with the enemies of the past and restoring pride as a collective. The leader aided by 'transference' may tap into the processes of the unconscious to mobilize the masses. In the context of the role of the charismatic leader, Fromm

(1982) points towards an avenue to explore, "The transference phenomenon, namely the voluntary dependence of a person on other persons in authority, a situation in which a person feels helpless, in need of a leader of stronger authority, ready to submit to this authority, is one of the most frequent and most important phenomena in social life, quite beyond the individual family and analytical situation. Anybody who is willing to see can discover the tremendous role that transference plays socially, politically and in religious life" (p. 41). Picking up moments of triumph from historical events – termed "chosen glory" by Volkan (2013) does not seem to work as well to restore a sense of pride of the group.

Processing injury and loss

Freud (1917 [1915]) speaking of the process of mourning observes "Each single one of the memories and expectations in which the libido is bound to the object is brought up and hyper-cathected and detachment of the libido is accomplished in respect of it. Why this compromise with the command of reality is carried out piecemeal should be so extraordinarily painful is not at all easy to explain in terms of economics. It is remarkable that this painful unpleasure is taken as a matter of course by us. The fact, is however, when the work of mourning is completed the ego becomes free and uninhibited again" (p. 245).

In the context of the Vietnam Veterans Memorial in Washington D.C. as an expression of mourning for the loss of American lives in the Vietnam War, Volkan, V (1997) illustrates the process of mourning with regard to large traumatic events and quotes Volkan, K (1992), senior editor in the Middle East Times: "As a reflection of death the memorial allows the living to fuse with the dead, through sight and touch. As a reflection of the psychodynamics of mourning, Lin's creativity resulted in a ritual that is soothing in itself; visitors symbolically repeat the mourning process, and thus master it, every time they come and go, touch the stone and leave."

The visitors read the names of the dead, with the granite walls reflecting their own image and can use pencil and paper to get a silhouette of the name and take is as a concrete material remembrance evoking memories, associations and feelings. Malhotra, 2018 writes "This was the first time that the importance of material memory truly dawned on me- the ability of an object or possession to retain memory and act as a stimulus for recollection" (p. 4).

Partition Museum, Amritsar in India

The Partition Museum in Amritsar, in the Indian side of Punjab, was opened in August 2017 to remember all those millions who lost their homes or loved ones at the time India was divided into the two separate entities of India and Pakistan in 1947. It is a pioneering attempt as part of the process of acknowledging and initiating the process of mourning with regard to the feelings of loss and trauma.

The Partition Museum is conceptualized as a *People's Museum* and thousands of people who have shared their histories and artefacts. The Museum has oral histories, soundscape in each gallery, original artefacts donated by refugees, newspapers, magazines and photographs showing the migration and camps, letters written by refugees, government documents as well as art installations. Malhotra (2022) talks about two objects a metallic vessel – *ghara* and a yardstick – *gaz* – which had travelled from Lahore to Amritsar and then Delhi in her family and writes "And when they were picked up, grazed, studied, remembered and situated in anecdotes of a time gone by, they proved to be the most effortless yet effective stimulus for extracting memory" (p. 4).[4]

Group processes

In individual therapy, awareness of unconscious intra-psychic processes of splitting and projection is used to help a person acknowledge and accept the disowned split 'bad' parts and take back the projections on to 'other' figures.

It would be constructive to initiate group processes of accessing, acknowledging and articulating the emotions aroused by the 'bad' parts, thus making them more manageable. This effort is essential to help moving towards accepting, owning up and learning to take responsibility at a collective level and take back projections made on to the 'other' community. Some of the key components of the process to move towards better inter-community relations are: developing and fine-tuning the process of the application of psychoanalytical tools to group dynamics; applying the understandings of the play of intra- and inter-psychic processes; developing tools and strategies to initiate group processes towards acceptance of the good and bad aspects of itself by a community. This could in the longer term enable a shift to a healthier middle state instead of extreme swings between the 'good' and the 'bad', between 'idealization' and 'persecution' both at an individual and collective level.

Notes

1 https://indianexpress.com/article/india/manipur-violence-meitei-kuki-tribe-conflict-four-months-8956725/

2 Laws and Decrees Timeline Layer. United States Holocaust Museum. https://www.ushmm.org/m/pdfs/20180228_3_Laws_and_Decrees_Timeline.pptx.pdf. Retrieved 23 March 2022.

3 In 1867, Canada instituted a policy of Aboriginal assimilation designed to transform communities from "savage" to "civilized." Canadian law forced Aboriginal parents under threat of prosecution to send their children to the schools. https://trauma-informed.ca/trauma-and-first-nations-people/residential-chools/#:~:text=In%201867%2C%20Canada%20instituted%20a,their%20children%20to%20the%20schools. Retrieved 1 6 June 2022.

4 For a digital repository of material culture from the Indian subcontinent, see: https://museumofmaterialmemory.com/

Bibliography

Arendt, Hannah. 1951. The Origins of Totalitarianism. London: Penguin Modern Classics.
Bacchetta, P. 2004. Gender in the Hindu Nation, RSS Women as Ideologues. New Delhi. Women Unlimited (an associate of Kali for Women).
Dohnanyi, Klaus Von, Mayor of the Free and Hanseactic City of Hamburg. Opening Ceremony: 34th IPA Congress, Hamburg, 1985 on Sunday 28 July 1985. 1986). International Journal of Psycho-Analysis, Vol. 67, pp. 3–8.
Erikson, E. H. 1966. D. Ontogeny of ritualization. Ontogeny of ritualization in man. Philosophical Transactions of the Royal Society B, Vol. 251, No. 772, pp. 337–349.
Freud, S. 1917[1915]. Mourning and melancholia. Standard Edition,
Freud S. 1921. Group psychology and the analysis of the ego. Standard Edition XVIII.
Freud S. 1930[1929]. Civilization and its Discontents. Standard Edition XXI.
Fromm. E. 1982. Greatness and Limitations of Freud's Thought. Abacus. London.
Jacques, Elliot. 1955. Social systems as defence against persecutory and depressive anxiety: a contribution to the psycho-analytical study of social processes. In M. Klein, P. Heimann and R. Money-Kyrle (eds) New Directions in Psycho-Analysis. London. Tavistock.
Jost John T., Glaser Jack, Kruglanski, Arie W and Sulloway, Frank J. 2003. 'Political Conservatism as Motivated Social Cognition', Psychological Bulletin, Vol. 129, No. 3, pp. 339–375.
Kakar, Sudhir. 1995. The Colours of Violence. Gurugram, Haryana: Viking, Penguin Books India.
Kernberg, Otto. 1995. Borderline Conditions and Pathological Narcissism. The Masterwork Series. file:///E:/Psychoanalysis%202/Books/(The%20Master%20Work%20Series)%20Otto%20F.%20Kernberg%20-%20Borderline%20Conditions%20and%20Pathological%20Narcissism-Jason%20Aronson,%20Inc.%20(2000).pdf
Koonz, Claudia. 1987. Mothers in the Fatherland. New York: St. Martin's Press.
Malhotra, A. 2018. Remnants of a Separation – A History of the Partition Through Material Memory. Gurugram, Haryana: HarperCollins Publishers India.
Malhotra, A. 2022. In the Language of Remembering – The Inheritance of Partition. Gurugram, Haryana: HarperCollins Publishers India.
Mitscherlich, A. 1971. Psychoanalysis and Aggression in Large Groups. International Journal of Psychoanalysis, Vol. 52, p. 161
Parker, A. et al. (eds). 1992. Nationalisms and Sexualities. New York: Routledge.
Pash, A.S.S. Sabse khatarnak kya hota hai. https://ncert.nic.in/textbook/pdf/khar119.pdf. Retrieved 8th June 2022.
Rosencranz, M.S. Halina. 2015. Group Work with Holocaust Survivors and Descendants (claimscon.org). Retrieved 16th June 2022.
Stalin. K. 2007. India Untouched – Stories of a People Apart. Documentary Film.
Volkan, V. 1986. The narcissism of minor differences in the psychological gap between nations. Psychoanalytic Inquiry. 1986/01 Vol. 6, No. 2.
Volkan, V. 1997. Bloodlines – From Ethnic Pride to Ethnic Terrorism. Boulder, Colorado: Westview Press.
Volkan, V. 2009. Large Group Identity, International Relations and Psychoanalysis. International Forum of Psychoanalysis, Vol. 18, No. 4, pp. 206–213.
Volkan, V. 2013. Large Group-Psychology in its Own Right: Large Group Identity & Peace Making. International Journal of Applied Psychoanalytic Studies, Vol. 10, No. 3, pp. 210–246.
Yengde, S. 2019. Caste Matters. New Delhi: Penguin-Viking.

7 Masculinity and Authoritarianism in India[1]

Introduction

The novel corona virus pandemic in India cutting across class, race, religion, ethnicity and nationality has exacerbated the process of demonizing the "other." The coining of the term "Corona Jihad" in popular discourse, implying the use of biological warfare suicide virus bombers to spread death, is indicative of the nature of politics of polarization at play. The headlines of articles in publications illustrate the dynamics and speak for themselves—"BJP's Karnataka MP calls Delhi's Tablighi Jamaat event 'corona jihad'[2]; 'Tablighi Jamaat members should be killed by firing bullets: MNS Chief Raj Thackerey'[3] and 'Half of India's Covid cases below the age of 40, a third linked to Talbighi Jamaat': Govt."[4]

An international gathering of the Islamic organization "Talbighi Jamaat" was held in mid-March 2020 at Hazrat Nizamuddin in Delhi with the knowledge of and with all due permissions of the authorities. This gathering is believed to have contributed to the rapid spread of the corona virus after participants at the gathering who dispersed to various parts of the country tested positive. These circumstances provided a convenient peg to the divisiveness being stoked in the country.

The polarization heightened by the Covid-19 virus is on a continuum of dynamics at play before the arrival of the pandemic. In a first for India, the ruling Bharatiya Janata Party (BJP) Government brought in a law discriminating on the ground of religion—the Citizen Amendment Act, 2019. This led to massive protests in several parts of the country.[5] The communal polarization was stoked by the ruling dispensation leading to riots in Delhi, the capital of India, in February 2020. The preventive steps to contain the corona pandemic saw the use of coercive police force and the breaking up of protests against the discriminatory law.

The arena for the full play of polarizing politics was set by the massive verdict of the 2019 elections to the Indian Parliament in favour of muscular nationalism and the "roaring lion son of Mother India" in the shape of celibate Prime Minister, Narendra Modi. Economic factors like increasing unemployment, farmers' distress, hardships caused by demonetization and

DOI: 10.4324/9781003626794-8

the newly introduced Goods and Services Tax, seem to have got trumped in one fell stroke by "surgical strikes" into Pakistani territory by Indian Armed Forces and is believed to have contributed to the 2019 electoral sweep of the hypernationalist BJP.

Psyche and society

Like a prism that reveals a spectrum of colours of apparently white light, the psychoanalytical angle of viewing is not an attempt to put forth a single factor explanation, but to add a perhaps hidden dimension of the psyche to the nature of the possible dynamics at play, which may have contributed to the landslide victory of an authoritarian party. There is a trend in the rise of aggressive triumphant leaders the world over, and each society will have certain facets that feed into the appeal of the virile strong man. Acknowledging the contribution of psychoanalysis to understanding individual mental health, the present work attempts to go beyond the individual psyche and apply a psychoanalytic approach to social issues. My views on these matters have evolved through almost four decades of involvement with social organizations and movements working for radical social change, as well as dealing with the numerous obstacles to achieving social change, such as a reluctance to acknowledge the psychological dimensions to social problems. Another possible reason for the marginalization of the need to redefine relationships is ignoring psychological needs within organizations working for a more egalitarian society.

About half a century after Karl Marx, Sigmund Freud evolved the analytical tools to understand the individual's unconscious drives to power and dominance. Firstly, a synthesis of Marx and Freud might have helped Marx's votaries to check tendencies of dominance within their own organizations. Second is the lack of attention to the irrational factors at play while trying to tackle broad phenomena whether of militant nationalism, religious fanaticism, xenophobia, or fascism. Adorno, Frenkel-Brunswik, Levinson and Sanford (1950) based on extensive research post-World War II (WWII) into personality structure and susceptibility to anti-democratic ideology in the United States speaking of Fascism say "Since by its very nature it favours the few at the expense of the many, it cannot possibly demonstrate that it will so improve the situation of most people that their real interests will be served. It must therefore make its major appeal, not to rational self-interest, but to emotional needs—often to the most primitive and irrational wishes and fears" (p. 10). Twemlow and Parens (2006) advance the view that Freud's main legacy will be the application of psychoanalysis to community and social problems and strongly advocate community psychoanalysis. In the same vein, Boheleber (2010) notes, "Although, for Freud, the clinical realm was the matrix from which psychoanalysis evolved, he always regarded psychoanalysis as more than a therapeutic method. In his understanding, its purview extended to the analytic investigation of cultural phenomena and the consequences of social disasters" (p. xv).

Despite social diversity, there is universality to certain aspects of the psyche which an ideology like fascism utilizes. Anxieties, insecurities, feelings of rage and anger are part of daily human existence. Alongside are positive feelings of belonging to a community, of love for the land they inhabit and for fellow human beings. While positive and negative feelings can acquire a social face, it is the interface of politics and psychoanalysis that can determine how both negative and positive feelings in the psyche become mobilized for a fascist agenda. Furthermore, the working of the psyche of an individual appears distinct from that of the individual functioning as part of a group. Taking the thread further, Boheleber (2010) observes that the phenomenon of anti-Semitism requires an interdisciplinary approach and speaking of the role of psychoanalysis writes, "This, however, does not impair its ability to trace back the attraction exerted by ideologies and nationalist/ethnic phantasms and the extraordinarily strong affects associated with them to unconscious factors and to provide psychological explanations for them" (p. 161).

Literature review

As far back as in 1895, Le Bon in *Psychologie des foules* translated into English in 1896 as "The Crowd: A Study of the Popular Mind" articulated some universal aspects of the psyche: "We see, then, that the disappearance of the conscious personality, the predominance of the unconscious personality, the turning by means of suggestion and contagion of feelings and ideas in an identical direction, the tendency to immediately transform the suggested ideas into acts; these we see, are the principal characteristics of the individual forming part of the group" (Le Bon, 1896, p. 12). Le Bon goes on to mention certain other characteristics of group functioning, which are worth extracting: "The simplicity and exaggeration of crowds have for result, that a throng knows neither doubt or uncertainty. …A suspicion transforms itself as soon as announced into incontrovertible evidence. A commencement of antipathy or disapprobation, which in the case of an individual would not gain strength, becomes at once furious hatred in the case of an individual in a crowd" (Le Bon, 1896, p. 35).

Speaking of a "fascist state of mind," Bollas (1992) says, "Doubt, uncertainty, self-interrogation, are equivalent to weakness and must be expelled from the mind to maintain ideological certainty. This is accompanied by a special act of binding as doubts and counter-views are expelled, and the mind ceases to be complex, achieving a simplicity held together initially by bindings around the signs of the ideology. Political slogans, ideological maxims, oaths, material icons fill the gap previously occupied by the polysemousness of the symbolic order" (p. 201).

Likewise, McDougall in "The Group Mind" (1920) describes the functioning of a group as "excessively emotional, impulsive, violent, fickle, inconsistent, irresolute and extreme in action, displaying only the coarser emotions and the less refined sentiments, extremely suggestible, careless in deliberation, hasty in judgment, incapable of any but the simpler and imperfect forms of reasoning; easily swayed and led ... and apt to be carried away by the consciousness of its own force, so that it tends to produce all the manifestations we have learned to expect of any irresponsible and absolute power" (p. 45).

Akhtar (2005) speaking of the appeal of fundamentalism observes that it offers "Instead of complexity–simplicity, instead of uncertainty–certainty, instead of moral ambiguity–moral clarity, instead of impurity–purity. We are pure people. We are pure Hindus, we are pure Muslims, we are pure Jews, we are pure Christians. Keep others away from us; don't let others mess this up. Don't let the *mlecchas* come near us, we are pure Brahmins.

Then, instead of personal responsibility, of conduct, of life, where a person says I am responsible for what I am saying, doing, how I am behaving; my sex life, my hostile life, my greedy life, my financial life is my business and my responsibility. I take responsibility for what I am doing and what I have done to others and to myself. The fundamentalist says don't worry, we will take over responsibility, we will show you how to kill Muslims, don't worry. The fundamentalist takes over responsibility and says you are not responsible for your conduct, we are responsible. This relieves one of personal responsibility."

It is Wilfred Bion who proposed the thesis that when isolated individuals come together in groups, their anxiety mobilizes collective psychotic defences to stabilize and reassure themselves. He went on to propose a conception of unconscious group collusion that offers a bridge between the seeming disjunct between individual and group functioning. According to Bion (1955), "The apparent difference between group psychology and individual psychology is an illusion produced by the fact that the group brings into prominence phenomena which appear alien to an observer unaccustomed to using the group" (p. 461). Bion effectively draws from and builds upon Kleinian theory in the arena of group functioning. "I think that the central position in group dynamics is occupied by the more primitive mechanisms which Melanie Klein has described as peculiar to the paranoid-schizoid and depressive positions. [...] it is not simply a matter of the incompleteness of the illumination provided by Freud's discovery of the family group as the prototype of all groups, but the fact that this incompleteness leaves out the source of the main emotional drives of the group" (p. 475).

Segal's exposition of the primitive anxieties generated in the paranoid-schizoid position can be applied to the context of Hindu–Muslim relations in India. Segal (1957) says, "...the paranoid-schizoid position anxieties of a primitive nature threaten the immature ego and lead to a mobilization of primitive defenses. Splitting, idealization and projective identification operate to create rudimentary structures made up of idealized good objects kept far apart from persecuting bad ones. The individual's own impulses are similarly split and he directs all his love toward the good object and all his hatred against the bad one. As a consequence of the projection, the leading anxiety is paranoid, and the preoccupation is with survival of the self."

In the context of linking religion and nationalism, Nandy (2016) analyses the role played and the impact on Hindu–Muslim relations by the partition of 1947, which led to the birth of two independent countries, India and Pakistan. He observes "It is very strange that in South Asia, both, the leader of the Hindus, who produced the Bible of Hindu nationalism—Vinayak Damodar Savarkar, and the leader of Muslim nationalism who carved out a Muslim state in the subcontinent, Pakistan—Mohammad Ali Jinnah, were non religious. And both had a deep contempt for ordinary Hindus and ordinary Muslims. But both felt that we must follow the European pattern and have proper nation-states, and to have proper nation-states you have to have nationalities.

Contempt for Hindus and Muslims is writ large in the lives and the writings of these two champions—Jinnah and Savarkar. An important part of the story is that this was an attempt to engineer an entire religious community into a nationality, and it produced nothing of the sort, but in the process divided the two communities and created permanent tension between the two. It is a bit like what happened in Palestine. But one should not forget that relations between Jews and Muslims virtually everywhere, in the Maghreb, in the Ottoman Empire, in Moorish Spain, were better than in the rest of Europe. But today, they are fighting like cats and dogs and this bitterness has lasted in Israel/Palestine for sixty-five years and in South Asia (India/Pakistan) for sixty-five years, because the political processes in both places incurred this bitterness."

Boheleber (2010) in the context of anti-Semitism enmeshing with Nationalism in Germany makes an invaluable contribution with regard to unconscious phantasies, which get activated and channelized—"The unconscious fantasies I have derived from the sensationalist and anti-Semitic notions revolve around ideal states (a) being the only one to receive maternal affection and care and eliminating rivals; (b) participating in an ideal, pure state undisturbed by any kind of otherness; (c) merging with and being assimilated into an organic whole, which is unconsciously imagined as restoration of the union with the maternal primary object and felt to be the overcoming of an individual, split-off, and alienated existence" (pp. 173–174).

Uncovering the links between the processes of the unconscious and the dynamics of mobilization of individuals may open up fruitful conversations in the engagement with fascism.

Present exploration

I set out by attempting to give shape to the abstract processes of group psychology in the specific situation of present-day India. Next, I attempt to unravel the link between the individual psyche and behaviour in a group. In the instances of communal violence and killings in India, there have been instances of violence by the minority Muslim community, but predominantly the perpetrators have been Hindu men, who are therefore an important focus for this exploration. Undoubtedly, there is fascist–fundamentalist stream in the Muslim polity in India, which in many ways feeds into Hindu fascist-fundamentalism; however, majoritarian fundamentalism is more dangerous, as evidenced by the incidents of communal violence and lynching against minority communities. Finally, I attempt to explore factors, predominantly unconscious, in the Indian Hindu male psyche,[6] which I believe operate in the mobilization for a fascist–fundamentalist agenda.

At a rational plane, successful polarization of society can ensure an electoral win based solely on the Hindu majority vote and is indicative of the deep roots and dangers posed by fascism in India. The BJP is the political formation, which fights elections and is the current ruling party. It is one of a number of organizations collectively referred to as the "Sangh Parivar" or "Collective Family." The beginning was made by the founding of the Rashtriya Swayamsevak Sangh (RSS) in 1925. The organization thereafter formed organizations to work among various sections of society—the Rashtriya Sevika Samiti for women, the Akhil Bharatiya Vidyarthi Parishad for students, the Bharatiya Mazdoor Sangh for workers, the Akhil Bharatiya Adhivakta Sangh for lawyers, the religious organization Vishva Hindu Parishad, the militant Hindu group Bajrang Dal and the farmers' union Bharatiya Kisan Sangh, among others. "Hindutva" is the term used for the monolithic, aggressive, violent form of the type of Hinduism advocated by right-wing fascist formations and constitutes the ideological underpinning of all these formations.

In the context of distinguishing the Hindu religion from "Hindutva," Nandy's (2016) observation based on a study of the massacres at the time of the partition of India in 1947 is illuminating "It was a surprise to see that those who resisted the violence, and there were very many of them, invoked their religion to do so. They believed that those who killed were actually flouting the principles of their religion and, as devout Hindus or devout Muslims, they all did it to protect their neighbours belonging to other religions."

Parliamentary democracy and elections are but one of the many instrumentalities used for the propagation and perpetuation of the ideology. Electoral victory by the Hindutva lobby, through communal polarization of the polity (as in the Gujarat assembly elections after the 2002 massacres of Muslims), is but a byproduct of the process of mobilization, and not an end in itself. Following 28 February 2007, burning of two compartments of a train full of Hindu "*kar-sevaks*" (people who had volunteered to build a Ram temple at the site of the demolished Babri Masjid[7] in Ayodhya) and the death of about 60 persons in Godhra, Gujarat, retaliatory violence against Muslims in Gujarat began. Extensive killings and rapes of Muslims immediately followed with a complicit BJP State Government. About 2000 Muslims are believed to have died in the carnage, believed to be pre-meditated and not a spontaneous reaction to the train burning. Several independent investigations into the atrocities brought out these facts of a pre-planned anti-Muslim pogrom.[8]

Hindus form the majority population in India, and Muslims constitute the largest majority at about 14% of the population (Census of India 2011). Yet, ever since the carving out of a Muslim majority Pakistan and the birth of independent India in 1947, the Hindu fear of being attacked, outnumbered and annihilated by the Muslims has played a key role in the mobilization of Hindus for attacking the community. The success of a Joseph Goebbels-like propaganda and the implanting of irrational beliefs in the Hindu community, such as "Hindus are being persecuted in their own country," "Muslims have four wives and 64 children," "Hindus will soon be a minority in India" or "More Hindus are killed in riots," probably reinforce the splitting, idealization and projective identification operating in the psyche. Such propaganda has been systematically carried out in all sectors of society by all the wings of the "Sangh Parivar."

The dynamics spelt out by Le Bon, Mc Dougal and Bollas are at full play in the social and political arena in India. The imagery of battle in the minds of people is generally not amenable to logic or rationality. For example, attackers like Taimur[9] and Genghis Khan,[10] who invaded and looted India several centuries ago, are conflated with present-day Indian Muslims in order to exploit existing antipathies between Hindus and Muslims and turn it into full-blown "othering" of the Muslim community as the repository of all evil. In the context of the Serb–Bosnian conflict, Volkan (1997) describes in detail the invocation by Slobodan Milosevic of the historical trauma of Serbian defeat in the Battle of Kosovo in 1389 by the Ottoman Empire and the conflation of the present Bosnian Muslims with Ottoman Turks.

Common threads of fascism

Although there is no unifying political doctrine associated with fascism, the shared features of fascist movements include: aggressive and unquestioning nationalism; belief in the supremacy of one national, ethnic or religious group over others; disrespect for democratic and liberal institutions, even as they are used to attain power; a profound hatred for socialism; insistence on obedience to a powerful and absolute leader; and a strong association with militarism and a demagogic approach that appeals to and whips up the basest emotions in a mob, making it suggestible, hasty in judgment, easily swayed and carried away by the consciousness of its own force.[11]

It is these features of the Hindutva movement, spearheaded by the RSS, that permit comparisons with the Partito Nazionale Fascista (PNF) founded by Benito Mussolini, Oswald Mosley's Blackshirts in Britain, the Iron Guard in Romania, the Croix de Feuin France and the Nazi Party in Germany.

The Sangh has a rigidly hierarchical structure, with nominated leaders and the *Sarsanghachalak* as the "Supreme Commander." Though the Sangh is open to married men, the *grihastha* (householder) is on a lower footing than the *brahmachari*, the virile but celibate son of Bharat Mata (Mother India) embodied in the *pracharak* (preacher). RSS ideologue Madhav Sadashiv Golwalkar (1939) in "We or our Nationhood Defined," professed great appreciation for the Nazi ideology and substituted the valorized German "nation" with the desired Hindu "nation" and Muslims in place of the Jews. Not much has changed since Golwalkar's time. The underpinning ideology of the organization continues to be based on the notion of a weakening Hindu race due to the pernicious influence of others.

Since its formation in 1925, it has been the Rashtriya Swayam Sevak's agenda to transform a relatively pluralistic and liberal Hinduism into an aggressive Hindutva, with a call to attack minorities. While Christians have also been targeted by Hindutva forces, special virulence is reserved for Muslims. As Kakar (1995) puts it—"There is a special quality to the enmity I feel for a person who resembles me but is not me. Next to my brother, it is my neighbor the Ten Commandments enjoin me to love as I do myself, precisely because my neighbor is the one I am most likely to consider as a rival" (p. 55).

One can take the view that just as there are people who propagate capitalism, communism or socialism in society, there are people and groups who believe in and propagate fascism. Indeed, fascism in India would not be such a threat if it were confined to groups like the RSS and its affiliates. The situation becomes worrying when a sizable section of people starts subscribing to and implementing the fascist agenda. The widespread support to the fascist agenda was amply demonstrated by the large-scale killing of Muslims in Gujarat in February–March 2002 by mobs numbering 20,000–25,000 in places, predominantly with the general approval of Gujarat's Hindu community. The support also manifested itself in the State Assembly elections later that year and the "peoples' verdict" of returning the BJP Government to power in Gujarat. This "victory" was used extensively to silence critics by sledgehammering the idea that the "Sovereign-Supreme People" had spoken, demonstrating the triumph of democracy. In fact, after the successful completion of an almost 5-year term, the BJP using the earlier tested method of whipping up anti-Muslim sentiments also won all the subsequent elections to the Gujarat State Assembly in 2007, 2012 and

2017, clearly illustrating the deep division along communal–religious lines in the Gujarat polity.

Analytical explorations: Lure of fascism in India

A theoretical construct that posits the *Sangh Parivar* as fascists and refuses to see public support to fascist ideology cannot take us forward in developing insights crucial to combat the spread of fascism. Wilhelm Reich writing of the rise of fascism in Germany in the 1920s begins with the recognition that a large section of the working class in Germany supported fascism. The official explanation by the German Communist Party for this support did not lead to an understanding of the phenomenology of the support. Unfortunately, the anti-fascist, left and progressive forces in India, much like the Communist Party in Germany in the 1930s, spare scant thought to the complex factors in the individual psyche at play in the mobilization by the present-day fascist forces. Reich's pioneering work into the psyche of the "common man" or "little man" who is enslaved and craves for authority but who also has a converse side is relevant to contemporary India. The interconnections he draws between daily life, sexuality, family, work place and the growth of fascism can assist in understanding its proliferation in India in the past couple of decades.

It is to try and unravel what Foucault (1983) eloquently describes as: "… the fascism in us all, in our heads and in our everyday behaviour, the fascism that causes us to love power, to desire the very thing that dominates and exploits us" (p. xiii). The particularities of the psyche, which make it amenable/vulnerable or drawn to fascist ideologies, would vary in different societies. Here, I attempt to explore possible facets of the Hindu male psyche, which may make it prey to the "lure of fascism." The positioning of the classical Oedipal complex and its play in the upbringing and childhood of boys in India may be a fruitful pathway of enquiry. Analysing the impact of culture and departing from the presumed universality of textbook oedipal dynamics need not be looked upon as abandonment of Freudian psycho-analysis. In fact, Freud (1923) leaves space for an alternative resolution of the Oedipus complex: "Along with the demolition of the Oedipus complex, the boy's object-cathexis of his mother must be given up. Its place may be filled by one of two things: either identification with his mother or an intensification of his identification with the father. We are accustomed to regard the latter outcome as more normal; it permits the affectionate relation to the mother to be in a measure retained" (p. 32).

Sex and intimacy

The nature of relations between the husband and wife in India, as well as the role model for women as to what constitutes appreciation in society impacts the dynamics of the father–mother–son triad. It is likely that this remains true even for a large majority of modern young women in the big cities whose appearance, attire and behaviour seems far removed from women brought up in a conservative village or small town in India. Outward changes are not necessarily accompanied or reflected in the inner world where possibly the process of change follows a dynamic not clear to us but which appears to be definitely slower in pace. Roland (1989) writing of Indian Identity and colonialism comments, "To understand this is to recognize that while Ashish's father's values, lifestyle, and even manner of authority were overwhelmingly Western, the inner emotional structure of the father–son hierarchical relationship was totally Indian" (p. 31).

In a society of "arranged marriages" or matches arranged by families in accordance with rules of caste, kinship and class, the bride and the bridegroom are almost strangers to each other. After the ceremony, the much glamorized "*suhaag raat*" (wedding night) may at one end of the spectrum turn out to be practically bridal rape with implicit if not explicit societal approval and endorsement by the groom's mother. It is likely that in a number of cases, the groom, eagerly anticipating the "deflowering" of his "virgin bride," may not even take her feelings into account. In fact, the law pertaining to rape in India excludes marriage and sanctions the husband's sacrosanct privilege to sexual intercourse with his wife.

From these stark beginnings, the space for conjugal relations remains constricted in Indian society. Speaking of relations between the sexes, Kakar (1989) notes that "Physical love will tend to be a shame ridden affair, a sharp stabbing of lust with little love and even less passion" (p. 19). In fact, it appears that the clinics of the psychotherapists practicing in big cities do comprise of a sizable section of women depressed and/or disillusioned after marriage. Kakar's conclusions are however based not on observations about middle-and upper-middle class women who come for psychotherapy, but also on interviews with so-called lower-caste, poor women and portray a uniformly miserable picture with regard to relations between the sexes in marriage. The expressions used indicative of the prerogative of the male speak volumes with regard to the issue of satisfaction for the women in sexual relations, namely, "*Hafte mein ek bar lagwa lete hain*" (*trans.*: "I get it done to me once a week") (p. 22).

Given the lack of intimacy in marriage, the primary emotional centre of a woman is her children, especially the son. The son is something of a combination of a knight in shining armour or rescuer, as well as the repository of the mother's unfulfilled wishes. According to Kakar (1981), clinical experience consistently shows that, "displacement of a woman's sexual longings from her husband to her son poses one of the most difficult problems for a boy to handle" and "the surge of unbidden and uncontrollable affect seems to threaten to engulf him while at the same time it arouses acute anxiety." Kakar is speaking of individuals who had approached him for psychotherapy, seeking a constructive resolution. Roland (1989) based on psychoanalytically oriented therapeutic work in India writes, "Several women, quite psychologically sophisticated, have related to me that their husbands simply cannot tolerate too open assertiveness on their part because of unconsciously perceiving them as being so covertly powerful like their mothers. These women often give in to many of their husband's demands, some on rather important career issues, because to assert themselves would be to profoundly disturb the marital relationship—that is, the husband would begin to experience his wife as the powerful mother" (p. 152). Boheleber (2010) writes "*Xenophobia is fuelled by many fantasy systems, but, in ethnic conflicts, group fantasies invariably activate the unconscious fantasy of a powerful collective mother, providing security and sustenance on the one hand, but also capable of devouring and expulsion on the other*" (p. 167). It is possible, however, that these feelings of engulfment and anxiety aroused in the "boy-male" in some way get mobilized for an agenda of fascism and violence against the "other." In the next section, I attempt to explore these links.

Selfless sons

In the popular Indian epic Mahabharata, the patriarch Bhishma takes the course of embracing *brahmacharya* (celibacy) in his prime so that his father, the ruler of Hastinapur, can fulfil his desire of marrying a beautiful fisher girl. The bride's condition precedent to the marriage was that her children alone could lay claim to the throne, prompting Bhishma (a son by an earlier wife) to become celibate, thus ruling out the possibility of having heirs at all. In a similar vein, King Yayati is cursed by Sant Shukracharya to become old in his youth. The only way out is if his sons give him his youth. The elder sons refuse, while the youngest one exchanges his youth and is accorded honour and inherits the kingdom. Interestingly, Ramanujam (1999) points out that there are "very, very few stories of actual patricide in Hindu myth, literature and folklore" and that in the stories, generally "the son willingly gives up (often transfers) his political and sexual potency," in contrast to the Oedipal myth predicated on hostility of the son towards the father. Goldman (1978) speaking of Oedipal myths in Sanskrit epic literature writes, "What these stories show, however, is that in almost every case in which this struggle is worked out between a son and his actual father in the Sanskrit epic literature it is the latter who succeeds. Actual sons are, if good sons, passive to the point of self-destruction and are rewarded for their passivity and subservience. If they are bad, they are passively disobedient and are degraded as a punishment for their sins. The latter case, moreover, exists largely to serve as a contrast to the former. In neither case are they actually aggressive to their father, nor do they ever gain unimpeded access to the goals of maturity, independence and the free expression of sexuality."

In fact, there is little room for ambivalence towards parents. The role model imprinted on the psyche through innumerable folk-tales and mythology is that of an obedient son. The story of Shravan Kumar is a favourite tale exemplifying the dutiful son whose parents are old and unable to walk. However, as is prevalent practice in India, they want to want to go on a *"teerth-yatra"* (pilgrimage) in their old age. The *"teerths"* or pilgrimage centres were established across the length and breadth of India by ascetics of yore. Shravan Kumar carries both parents in a *"kanwar"*—something like a large-scale balance—with one parent in each of the pans with the bamboo pole across his shoulder. Shravan Kumar spends his youth trudging from one pilgrimage centre to another carrying his parents, proud to be of service to his parents and earns a lot of *"punya"* to his credit.

The denial of ambivalence in the mother–son dyad is expectedly standard fare of Hindi "Bollywood" films. However, the films of even progressive male directors reflect the denial of ambivalence. Films and popular media aside, the stories on which a child grows up emphasize the utter selflessness of the mother and total concern for the son with an underlying subtext of potential betrayal or doubt regarding the loyalty of the son, especially after marriage. A folktale from Uttar Pradesh in North India is worth recounting, as it makes the latent subtext manifest. A son gets married. The wife does not like her mother-in-law and there is constant antagonism and hostility. The wife asks her husband to cut out and get the heart of his mother. The son does the needful and is carrying the still beating heart of the mother in his hand. On the way, his toe bumps into a stone and he stumbles. The heart says, *"Beta chot to nahi ayi"* (*trans*: "Son, hope you were not hurt"). The emotive impact and the imprint left on the psyche by such stories are strong, more so when related in the mother tongue by the caregivers of the child.

Valorizing celibacy

The renouncing of sexual life by young men is reified by other cultural beliefs regarding loss of strength by the falling of the seed. The valorization of *brahmacharya* (celibacy) is taken to incredible lengths in Hindu religion. Thus, religious texts are replete with statements like, "*Brahmacharya* is so powerful that by strictly following it one can win over death." As Alter (1992) puts it: "A wrestler must not only abstain from sex, he must also build up his stock of semen and ensure that once built up it is as potent and strong as it can possibly be. The basis for this preoccupation is a belief that physical, personal, and intellectual strength emanates from semen. Semen is the locus of a person's moral character and physical prowess."

In fact, Bhishma Pitamaha, the patriarch of the epic Mahabharata as a result of being a dedicated *brahmachari* (celibate) was granted the boon of death-at-will and the power to change the course history of Hastinapur. These conceptions, however, are not only part of a mythical past but remain present-day beliefs. Sri Asaram Bapu, a contemporary religious guru with a sizable following, claims that sex is not a healthy activity. Asaramji, after bemoaning the pernicious influence of Dr. Sigmund Freud, attempts to harness the prestige of medical science to tradition and enjoins his followers to follow one Dr. Molvil Keith, MD who declares: "This seed (semen) is marrow to your bones, food to your brains, oil to your joints and sweetness to your breath and if you are a man, you should never lose a drop of it till you are thirty years of age and then only for the purpose of having a child which shall be blessed by heaven" (*The Times of India*, September 29, 2000). With the increase in the legal age of marriage and age of consent, adolescent boys in India have few socially acceptable outlets for their sexual drives.

Reverence of *brahmacharya* along with beliefs about loss of semen leading to weakness of the body, mind and spirit acts as a block to masturbation. Even when "indulged" in, it comes ridden with guilt, anxieties and fears about the consequences. On the other hand, "mother******" and "sister-******" are the commonest abuses and are part of routine speech across the country. In fact, interventions in incidents of harassment of women in public spaces often take the shape of abusing the perpetrator as "Sister******" while simultaneously trying to make him feel ashamed by enquiring whether he does not have mothers and sisters at home, in a way encapsulating the contradictory feelings of Indian males towards women in their family. The rigid incest taboo in India, like in most societies, is indicative of the need to prohibit sexual feelings towards family members, which are regarded as "un-brotherly" and "non-son-like" vis-à-vis boys/men and their mothers and sisters. These feelings for the "pure" mother and "virgin" sister evoke strong feelings of guilt and remorse. Sexual fantasies involving close family members along with lack of interaction and sexual activity among peers fuel further frustration accompanied by feelings of guilt and perversion. Thus, the suppression of sexuality, the intimate mother–son bond along with powerful images of powerful decapitating "Kali"(commonly depicted dancing nude with a garland of human skulls and holding a severed head in one of several hands gripping various weapons), and the son giving up his potency to his father is the mixed bag of the Indian male psyche. Kakar (1997) posits that in Indian society, rather than conflict, the son seems to require an Oedipal alliance with the father for autonomy vis-à-vis the mother and terms it "Maternal Enthrallment."

In fact, two vignettes from Kakar (1997) are worth recounting: "Mohan, too, we saw, became passionless whenever the motherly woman he fancied in the bus turned to face him. But instead of celibacy, he tried to hold onto desire by killing the sexual part of the mother, deadening the lower portion of her trunk, which threatened him with impotence. Furthermore, the imagined sexual overpowering of the mother, in the face of which the child feels hopelessly inadequate, with fears of being engulfed and swallowed by her dark depth, is not experienced by Mohan in the form of clear-cut fantasies but in a recurrent nightmare from which he wakes up screaming" (p. 68).

The second vignette seems illustrative of the father–boss–fuehrer interconnection: "He compared himself to a frightened mouse in the presence of his father and felt that this trait had persisted all through his life. If anyone argues loudly, he said, especially, my boss, I have to agree and cannot say what I believe to be true. In these sessions it became clear that Deven's fear of his father had largely to do with his sexual impulses. Whenever he talked of his attraction toward some girl or of his masturbation, it was in a very low, 'mouse-like' voice which I could hardly hear and this happened almost always at the end of the session when he could get away quickly. After any such confession, he would close his eyes tightly, clasp his hands on his stomach in an attitude of praying and cross his legs, as if protecting his genitals from retaliation" (p. 78).

An ingredient, which holds vital importance for our purposes, comes from the "Father" of Indian Psychoanalysis, Girendrasekhar Bose (the moving spirit behind the formation of the Indian Psychoanalytic Association in 1922): "The respectability of the mother image is sought to be neutralized by the substitution of the mother by the sister or women of lower social status and even prostitutes. *There is impaired potency and obsessional fear of not being able to satisfy the woman in the sexual act. The small penis complex receives a further strengthening from this source, the child's penis being considered too small for the mother*" (emphasis added) (1928).

Role of suppression of sexuality

This chapter is underpinned by the Reichian postulate that suppression of sexuality causes repression within the individual psyche and makes it a fertile ground for the spread of reactionary ideologies like fascism (carried forward by Deleuze and Guattari to the arena of the purpose served by Oedipalization of desire). The pioneering works of Kakar and Bose show the particularities and causative factors that contribute to the suppression of sexuality in Indian society. Observing that economic distress incites people to rebellion, while sexual distress prevents rebellion against both forms of suppression, Reich (1942) offers insights into the causative processes: "The moral inhibition of the child's natural sexuality, the last stage of which is the severe impairment of the child's genital sexuality, makes the child afraid, shy, fearful of authority, obedient, 'good', and 'docile' in the authoritarian sense of the word. It has a crippling effect on man's rebellious forces because every vital life impulse is now burdened with severe fear; and since sex is a forbidden subject, thought in general and man's critical faculty also become inhibited. In short, morality's aim is to produce acquiescent subjects who despite distress and humiliation are adjusted to the authoritarian order."

Deleuze and Guattari (1983) acknowledging the radical contribution of Reich, the first to posit sociological reasons for the suppression of sexuality by society and repression by the individual, write: "But social repression should not be understood by using as a starting point a familial repression coextensive with civilization—far from it; it must be civilization that must be understood in terms of social repression inherent to a given form of social production" (p. 129). Referring to the thesis of suppression of sexuality and sublimation as transcendent requirements for "Civilization," Reich in his inimitable manner remarks: "One becomes a bit sceptical and asks how is it possible for the masturbation of small children and the sexual intercourse of adolescents to disrupt the building of gas stations and the manufacturing of aeroplanes" (p. 63).

Deleuze and Guattari carry Reich's legacy forward and further the understanding of the role of suppression of sexuality in society: "It is therefore of vital importance for a society to repress desire, and even to find something more efficient than repression, so that repression, hierarchy, exploitation, and servitude are themselves desired. It is quite troublesome to say such rudimentary things: desire does not threaten society because it is a desire to sleep with the mother, but because it is revolutionary. And that does not at all mean that desire is something other than sexuality, but that sexuality and love do not live in the bedroom of Oedipus, they dream instead of wide open spaces, and cause strange flows to circulate that do not let themselves be stocked within an established order" (p. 127).

Self and individualism

If an understanding of the possible causes of the support to a fascist–fundamentalist ideology in the Hindu psyche, from the standpoint of theories around psychosexual stages of development, ego and super-ego development, object relations, psychosocial and narcissistic stages of development are carried out in a framework implicit with Western universalistic norms, it would result in viewing the Indian as well as other non-Western psyches as "inferior" or "distorted" with "pathological mothering" interfering with individuation and possibly more prey to fascism.

Obyesekere (2003) articulates the perspective of criticality towards the Western approach along with retaining sharpness towards one's own culture—"On the one hand, I'm very critical of the way European scholarship approaches the Other—you know, Third World cultures, including my own. I'm very critical of that. I'm also critical of my own culture particularly, and am terribly unpopular in Sri Lanka, at least among small groups of people, because I'm very critical of the nationalism in the country, the nationalism that led to this terrifying war in which we are now implicated and fortunately having a breathing spell right now" (p. 3).

While the sharpest manifestation of fascism in the last 100 years was undoubtedly in Europe, each society and culture engenders certain facets in the psyche, which can enmesh with a fascist ideology. As Roland (1989) writing of potentialities and pathologies in a society and culture from a cross-cultural psychological perspective puts it: "It is also apparent from clinical psychoanalytic work in India, Japan, and America that in each society there are distinct kinds of psychopathology, structural deficits, and unconscious conflicts—a finding that is generally congruent with anthropological work relating mental illness to specific cultural and social patterns" (p. 325).

An exploration towards an understanding of the processes at play in a mobilization for a fascist–fundamentalist agenda in India is not to make a case for individualism as a universal model of the self to be followed in all societies.[12] Acknowledging the more relational and contextual nature of the self in India as well as the effect of differential mothering on boundary formation between the self and others elaborated by Roland (1989), it is a plea for what could be called a middle path Indian self with slightly more space for autonomous functioning and for awareness, if not expression, of ambivalence and anger towards parents and elders in the family.

Roland's extremely empathetic view of the Indian self and sensitive work itself serves to illustrate the need for changes in this direction. Speaking of the we-self and multiple levels of communication of Indians, Roland (1989) writes: "A striking example of these different levels of communication is cited by Das (1976b): a man beat his wife in accordance with the complaints of his mother and sister, thus fulfilling structural hierarchical expectations within the family, but that night made love to her in such an indiscreet way that he clearly communicated to the others that his deeper loyalty and love was to his wife, not to his mother and sister. From reports of his wife, his mother and sister were crestfallen the next morning" (p. 222). Regardless of the contextualization of the Indian conscience rather than Universal norms, beating up a wife can hardly be looked upon as a healthy aspect of the male psyche and the marital relationship.

Roland's work also gives pointers to the role strong identification with family and community and the "we-self" of Indians can play in the "othering" of another community: "Strong identifications on the part of both women and men with their families and *jatis* (caste/community) often leads to feelings that others of another community may be tremendously different—which indeed they are in terms of customs, ethos, traditions and norms—whereas the inner psychological structures and modes of relationship may be overwhelmingly similar. The experiential sense of we-ness and we-self in the close identifications with one's own family and community thus enhances the perception of enormous differences in others" (pp. 225–226).

The prevalence of these processes across cultures is articulated by Boheleber in the context of Spitz's (1965) observations of the child's stranger anxiety in the preverbal period of object relationships: "In contrast, the pathological form of this relation seeks to exclude the stranger and to reassure oneself through a narcissistic mirroring in the mother. If a fantasy of homogeneity dominates at the level of the group, mirroring and self-reassurance take place in those group members who are like oneself. Ambivalence is unavoidable, however, and gives an aggressive charge to differences within the group, which must then be erased and projected outward. Such a world of narcissistic mirroring and purity results in massive persecutory aggression against those who are different and, thereby, threaten internal cohesion. This narcissism cannot tolerate the coexistence of anything different or deviant and has the tendency to become progressively more radical. Purity is only to be obtained through exclusion. In this way, belonging to an idealized, pure community and persecutory violence are closely connected and mutually dependent. In order keep the ideal of purity present, ever new impurities have to be found" (p. 196).

In a communally surcharged atmosphere, the role of the intense mother–son relationship in the context of the killing of people and rape of women from the "other" community with bordering on tacit approval is another area, which can be a fruitful direction of inquiry. Again, Roland gives some pointers in this direction, "A psychopathological dimension of this intense mother–son relationship tends to emerge when there are feelings of an omnipotent alliance on *both* sides; that is, both son and mother may have strong inner feelings of powerfulness with little or no constraints on what they want and/or should do as long as they feel deeply connected to each other" (p. 234).

It looks likely that colonialism meshed in with features present in the prevalent psyche and the aim of Macaulay[13] in setting up the education system in India to produce clerks resulted in the colourless "*babu*" (clerk) personality. This was again a mixed bag of worries about not getting employment, the single-track education system, family pressures to conform, marry, produce grandchildren and fulfil duties towards parents, which leaves little space to develop interests and healthy enjoyments. However, the anonymous, non-assertive, "nonentity" personality that gets pushed around in the workplace and takes the shape of the "obedient" son in the family has a converse authoritarian-negative side that gets mobilized in aid of the fascist–fundamentalist agenda. This agenda playing out in the sociopolitical arena enjoys sizable support of women. However, an analysis of the factors at play in the psyche of women, which enmesh with fascism in India, is outside the scope of the present work.

Protecting the mother

The notion of defending "our mothers and sisters" plays a core part in mobilization in an agenda of attacking the "enemy" community. Feelings of inadequacy, lack of potency symbolized in the small penis complex play another crucial role. The males of the "other" community are invariably looked upon as super-humanly virile, potent and lusting after our mothers and sisters. This is true of the view of black males by whites supremacists, Jews by Nazis as well as the viewing of Muslims by Hindu males.

In Gujarat long before any killings began, women's bodies were centrally used to successfully polarize the two communities. The rallying cry for large-scale mobilization of Hindus and for the first time of *Adivasis* (Indigenous peoples) was that, "They (Muslims) despoil our women!" Given the complicity of the state administration, the only hope of safety was in numbers and Muslims fled to areas where the community constituted a sizable proportion of the population. However, in Sanjeli village of Dahod district in Gujarat not one out of the 500 houses of Muslims comprising 40% of the population remains in the village. The "credit" for mobilizing about 25,000–30,000 *Adivasis* goes to Dilsukh *Maharaj*, himself a Bhil, who runs an ashram with a hostel for school children and is part of the *Sant Samaj* (Society of "sants-sanyasis," that is, individuals who have renounced the world). Dilsukh-ji declared that Muslims took "our" women and have "violated" at least 100 Bhil women in Sanjeli alone. Muslims, according to him, consider "our widows" to be everyone's property. Public meetings, speeches, pamphlets, schools, cultural groups, ashrams, philanthropic institutions, *babas, sants* and *maharajs* all have been systematically used as tools for the past decade by the "Sangh Parivar" to spread venom and demonize Muslims. After the Godhra train-burning incident on 27 February, rumours about Hindu women being abducted, raped and mutilated played a crucial role in the mobilization. Leading Gujarati language dailies like *Sandesh* and *Gujarat Samachar* carried headlines on 28 February–1 March 2002, like "10–15 Hindu women were dragged away by a fanatic mob from the railway compartment"; "Wicked villains of this mob kidnapped some ten women (*behno*– "sisters") whose whereabouts are not yet known"; "Helpless women were struggling to escape from the grip of *Saitans* (Devils)"; "Out of kidnapped young ladies from Sabarmati Express, dead bodies of two women recovered— breasts of women were cut off"—in flaming communal tension and feeding into righteous indignation and moral outrage providing a justification for the massacre and rape of Muslims that followed in the State. Psychoanalytically speaking, stories about breasts being cut off feed into associations of the nurturing breast of the mother being taken away, leading to intense feelings of infantile rage and anxiety, which can then get mobilized for channelization against the "enemy" community.

Building upon prevailing Hindu–Muslim antagonism, feeding into insecurities, stoking fears and the successful implanting of a belief that the majority Hindu community is under threat from the minority community lead to the crossing of a certain threshold where an "Othering" takes place. "Muslim" girls and women can never even be imagined as "mothers and sisters" of our "Hindu" boys. The stereotyping and boxing in of individual women into the categories of "whore" and "goddess" contributes to women of the other community being considered bitch-like and enjoying sex unlike the "dutiful" good woman. Simultaneously, the men of the "other" community get constructed as "animal-like" oversexed males lusting after and posing a threat to the women of "our" community.

The inaccurate conflation of invaders from the medieval period attacking "Mother India" and violating "pure" Hindu girls and women in the past with contemporary stories of Muslim men abducting, raping and mutilating our "mothers and sisters" leads to the successful demonizing of Muslims. Sexual violence against Muslim girls and women becomes a righteous moral act to save the "honor" of "our" mothers and sisters, at the same time emasculating the rapacious Muslim males and "dishonoring" the entire community.

The *Ram Janmabhoomi Rath Yatra* [Rally to Ram's birthplace in Ayodhya] seems to have played upon and crystallized the unconscious sense of humiliation in the Hindu psyche of the existence of Babri Masjid, as a phallic symbol that colonizes Mother India and emasculates the virile sons who failed to protect her, leading to the triumphant destruction of the Masjid by *kar-sevak*—volunteers in the service of Hindu religion. In a textbook illustration of what Volkan (1997) terms as "chosen trauma," Lal Krishna Advani, the leader of the BJP, at the time the main Opposition party in Parliament, started the Yatra from Somnath in 1992 invoking the plunder of the temple by Mahmud of Ghazni who invaded India and in 1025 AD looted the Somnath Temple and ended it at Babri Masjid. The destruction of the temple had nothing to do with Indian Muslims and in a masterful exercise at invoking past trauma as if it happened now leading to intensifying of emotions and justifiable anger against "them." The Yatra left a trail of riots and killings of Muslims in its wake.[14] The culmination in the demolition of the Masjid restored Hindu male virility and symbolic Hindu feminine purity (Bachcheta, 2004).

Conclusion

The idealization of the "pure" mother with no room for ambivalence, extreme suppression of sexuality, the revering of *brahmacharya*, the giving up of potency for father, the desire for a charismatic *fuhrer*—father who can be obeyed obviating the need for autonomous functioning and responsibility, the anxieties, frustrations and fears about virility along with the projection of all "negative," "impure," "lustful," "beast-like," onto the "Enemy Other" are possible areas of exploration, which may offer some insights and understandings of the processes at play and assist to devise strategies[15] to engage with a hate-ideology like fascism in India.

Notes

1 First published as "Aspects of male sexuality enmeshing with the rise of fascism in India: Tentative psychoanalytic explorations" in the International Journal of Applied Psychoanalytical Studies. Int J Appl Psychoanal Studies. 2020; 1–15.

2 https://theprint.in/politics/bjps-karnataka-mp-calls-delhis-tablighi-jamaat-event-corona-jihad/395511/

3 https://theprint.in/india/tablighi-jamaat-members-should-be-killed-by-firing-bullets-mns-chief-raj-thackeray/395270/

4 https://theprint.in/india/half-of-indias-covid-19-cases-below-the-age-of-40-a-third-linked-to-tablighi-jamaat-govt/395404/
5 See Shukla, R. (2020). Bubbling cauldron of hate–envy–fury: Playgrounds of splitting and projection. Int J Appl Psychoanal Studies, 17: 77-83. https://doi.org/10.1002/aps.1641
6 Given the impact of differences of caste, class, region, culture, social environment and individual upbringing in a country of subcontinental proportions, it is hazardous to posit an "Indian Hindu Male Psyche." The present use of the term for convenience is perhaps debatable and open to discussion.
7 The Babri Masjid was a mosque at Ayodhya in Faizabad district of Uttar Pradesh built by Mir Baqi, a general during the reign of Babar, the first Mughal Emperor. The "Sangh Parivar" comprised of Hindu nationalist organizations claimed that the mosque was built on the site of a temple marking the birthplace of the mythological hero "Lord Ram" after destroying the temple. They started a movement to reclaim the birthplace referred to as Ram Janmabhoomi. On 6 December 1992, the Babri Masjid was demolished by kar-sevaks (volunteers) at the culmination of the Ram Janmabhoomi Rath Yatra led by Lal Krishan Advani, leader of the BJP, the main opposition party in Parliament and the prime-ministerial candidate for the next General Elections in India to be held in 2009.
8 Harvest of Hatred—The Concerned Citizens 'Report on Gujarat, 2002, Manohar Books; "Maro! Kaapo! Balo!"—State, Society and Communalism in Gujarat, Peoples' Union for Democratic Rights (PUDR), May 2002; "We Have No Orders to Save You"—State Participation and Complicity in Communal Violence in Gujarat, April 2002, Human Rights Watch April 2002 Vol. 14, No. 3(C).
9 Taimur (1336–1405) also referred to as Tamerlane—Turkish King of Mongol descent who invaded India in 1398 and is said to have executed 100,000 captives, mostly Hindus in a single day.
10 Genghis Khan (1162–1227), founder of the Mongol Empire, born Temujin was declared "Khan" in 1206 and took the title "Genghis Khan." In 1221, he is said to have ravaged vast tracks of Punjab, attacked Multan and Lahore—his religion is speculated to be Shamanism or Tengriism prevalent in Mongol-Turkic tribes but he is inaccurately though widely perceived as a Muslim invader in India and in the mobilization for the killings of Muslims in Gujarat in 2002, slogans referring to Muslims as "Changez Khan ke aulad" (trans. Progeny of/Sired by Changez Khan) were extensively used to evoke murderous sentiments.
11 Chambers Dictionary of World History, 2003; Le Bon (1895).
12 Jack London (1876–1916)—Worker, Oyster Pirate, Railroad hobo, Prospector, Explorer, Author of "The Call of the Wild," "White Fang" and "The Sea Wolf" is an iconic example of unconfined individualism.
13 Lord Macaulay (1800–1859) set up the system of education in India, which remains the basic framework of teaching. Minutes on Indian Education delivered by Macaulay in 1835: "It is impossible for us, with our limited means, to attempt to educate the body of the people. We must at present do our best to form a class who may be interpreters between us and the millions whom we govern; a class of persons, Indian in blood and color, but English in taste, in opinions, in morals, and in intellect. To that class we may leave it to refine the vernacular dialects of the country, to enrich those dialects with terms of science borrowed from the Western nomenclature, and to render them by degrees fit vehicles for conveying knowledge to the great mass of the population."
14 https://www.indiatoday.in/magazine/cover-story/story/20091228-1990-l.k.-advanis-rath-yatra-chariot-of-fire-741621-2009-12-24. Retrieved 5 March 2020.
15 Learning to take responsibility for one's projections and taking them back at a collective level could be a possible direction of some form of community psychoanalysis.

Bibliography

Alter, J. S. (1992). The Wrestler's body, identity and ideology in North India, Berkeley, CA: University of California Press.

Bachcheta, P. (2004). Mother Goddesses and Warriors: RSS women as ideologues, Delhi, India: Women Unlimited.

Boheleber, W. (2010). Destructiveness, Intersubjectivity and Trauma: The Identity Crisis of Modern Psychoanalysis. London: Karnac.

Bollas, C. (1992). Being a Character, Psychoanalysis and Self Experience, New York, NY: Hill and Wang.

Bion, W. R. (1955). Group dynamics: A review. International Journal of Psycho-Analysis (vol. 33). Reprinted in M. Klein, P. Heimann, & R. Money-Kyrle (Eds.), New directions in psychoanalysis, London: Tavistock Publications, pp. 440–477, p. 457, 461, 475

Das, V. (1976b). Masks and faces: An essay on Punjabi Kinship. Contributions to Indian Sociology, Vol. 10, pp. 1–30.

Deleuze, G., & Guattari, F. (1983). Anti-Oedipus: Capitalism and Schizophrenia, Minneapolis, MN: University of Minnesota.

Freud, S. (1923). The ego and the Id Standard Edition XIX, Vol. 19. London: Hogarth Press.

Kakar, S. (1981). The inner world: A Psycho-Analytic Study of Childhood and Society in India, Delhi, India: OUP.

Kakar, S. (1989). Intimate Relations, Exploring Indian Sexuality, New Delhi, India: Penguin Books.

Kakar, S. (1995). The Colours of Violence, New Delhi, India: Penguin Books India.

Kakar, S. (1997). Culture and Psyche, Selected Essays, Delhi, India: OUP.

Le Bon, G. Psychology de foules. (1896). Translated English, The Crowd: A Study of the Popular Mind. New York: The Macmillan Co.

Nandy, A. (2016). Ashish Nandy: Why nationalism and secularism failed together, Chestnut Hill, MA: Reset Dialogues US. Retrieved from http://resetdoc.org/story/ashis-nandy-why-nationalism-and-secularism-failed-together/

Roland, A. (1989). In Search of Self in India and Japan, Toward a Cross-Cultural Psychology, Princeton, NJ: Princeton University Press.

Spitz, R. (1965). The First Year of Life: A Psychoanalytic Study of Normal and Deviant Development of Object Relations. New York, NY: International Universities.

Volkan, D. V. (1997). Bloodlines: From Ethnic Pride to Ethnic Terrorism, Boulder, CO: Westview Press.

Index

Note: Page numbers followed by "n" refer to notes.

For Product Safety Concerns and Information please contact our EU representative GPSR@taylorandfrancis.com Taylor & Francis Verlag GmbH, Kaufingerstraße 24, 80331 München, Germany

Batch number: 10799928

Printed by Printforce, the Netherlands